Springer Series on Advanced Practice Nursing

Terry T. Fulmer, PhD, C, FAAN, Series Editor
New York University School of Nursing

1993 Nurses, Nurse Practitioners: Evolution to Advanced Practice
Mathy D. Mezey, RN, EdD, FAAN, and Diane O. McGivern, RN, PhD, FAAN

1994 Nurse-Physician Collaboration: Care of Adults and the Elderly
Eugenia L. Siegler, MD, and Fay.W. Whitney, PhD, RN, FAAN

1995 Advanced Practice Nursing: A Guide to Professional Development
Mariah Snyder, PhD, RN, FAAN, and Michaelene Pheifer Mirr, RN, PhD, CS

1997 The Acute Care Practitioner
Barbara J. Daly, PhD, RN, FAAN

1997 Developing A Private Practice in Psychiatric Mental-Health Nursing
Susanne Fine, PhD, RN, CS

1998 Practice Issues for the Acute Care Nurse Practitioner
Ruth M. Kleinpell, PhD, RN, CCRN, and Mariann Piano, PhD, RN

Ruth M. Kleinpell, PhD, RN, ACNP, CCRN, received her diploma in nursing from Lutheran Medical Center School of Nursing, Cleveland, Ohio, and her baccalaureate, masters, and doctorate in nursing from University of Illinois College of Nursing Chicago, Illinois. Dr. Kleinpell received her Acute Care Nurse Practitioner at Rush University College of Nursing, Chicago, Illinois, and is certified as an Acute Care Nurse Practitioner. Dr. Kleinpell is a Teacher-Practitioner, Rush Presbyterian St. Luke's Medical Center and an Associate Professor at Rush University College of Nursing. Her clinical background is critical care nursing, and she is currently a faculty member in the Acute Care Nurse Practitioner program at Rush University College of Nursing. In 1996, Dr. Kleinpell received funding from the American Nurses Foundation to conduct research on ACNPs. Dr. Kleinpell has presented at national and international conferences and has published in the areas of critical care nursing, research, and advanced practice nursing.

Mariann R. Piano, PhD, RN, received her baccalaureate in nursing from Loyola University of Chicago and her masters and doctorate in nursing from University of Illinois College of Nursing, Chicago, Illinois. Dr. Piano is coordinator of the Critical Care Acute Care Nurse Practitioner program at the University of Illinois. Her clinical background is critical care nursing, and cardiovascular nursing. Dr. Piano has presented at national and international conferences and has published in the areas of cardiovascular physiology and pathophysiology and alcoholic heart muscle disease.

Practice Issues for the Acute Care Nurse Practitioner

Ruth M. Kleinpell, PhD, RN, CCRN
Mariann R. Piano, PhD, RN
Editors

Springer Publishing Company

Springer Publishing Company, Inc.
536 Broadway
New York, NY 10012-3955

Cover design by Janet Joachim
Acquisitions Editor: Ruth Chasek
Production Editor: Jeanne Libby

99 00 01 02 03 / 5 4 3 2 1

Library of Congress Cataloging-in-Publication Data

Practice issues for the acute care nurse practitioner / edited by Ruth M. Kleinpell and Mariann Piano.
p. cm.
Includes bibliographical references and index.
ISBN 0-8261-1204-8
1. Emergency nursing. 2. Intensive care nursing. 3. Nurse practitioners. I. Kleinpell, Ruth M. II. Piano, Mariann.
[DNLM: 1. Emergency Nursing. 2. Acute Disease—nursing. 3. Nurse Practitioners. WY 154P895 1998]
RT120.E4P72 1998
610.73'61—dc21
DNLM/DLC
for Library of Congress 98-27636
CIP

Printed in the United States of America

Contents

Foreword

Studies as early as the 1970s and extruding into the late 1980s have demonstrated repeatedly that nurse practitioners can provide cost-effective, high-quality primary care. The impetus and continued stimulus for the evolution of the nurse practitioner role has been in response to the lack of basic health services, particularly in rural and inner-city areas, where physicians did not want to practice. This shortage of adequate medical care to underserved and vulnerable populations, especially infants and children, opened the door to the spread of nurse practitioner programs from their start in Colorado to other parts of the country with similar physician supply problems. From the initial focus on health care for infants and children, nurse practitioner programs eventually expanded to include adults and the elderly, with their success assured as long as the need for primary care was evident and populations were available to be served.

As nurse practitioners established themselves as creditable providers of primary care, their role and their identity became nearly synonymous with primary care. In tthe late 1980s and ealry 1990s, another physician shortage was being identified, this time in the acute care settings. In some large hospitals, especially academic medical centers, the number of resident physicians was being reduced, leaving the hospitals with less manpower to keep up with the patient care demands of ever-increasing technology and higher patient acuity, spurred by shorter and shorter hospital stays. The logical response to this was the introduction of the nurse practitioner with specialized education in acute care medical management. Thus, the initiation of the Acute Care Nurse Practitioner (ACNP) movement.

These ACNPs are filling a different role than do their primary care counterparts in nursing. ACNPs work in both hospital and outpatient settings, they are employed by both physicians and health-care facilities, and they are both population- and unit-based. In spite of these multiple ways in which ACNPs actualize their roles, the unifying thread is that ACNPs manage patient care during some part of a patient's hospitalization. This fact alone requires that they work collaboratively with physicians to provide quality patient care. As more and more health-care facilities move into managed care, the economic benefit of using ACNPs becomes another factor that strengthens this role for nurses.

Beyond the educational materials available for ACNP students, very little has been written to support the practicing nurse in this relatively new advanced practice role. This book provides real world, practice-based information for the practicing ACNP. The editors and contributors to this book have provided current information on practice issues that should be valuable to all ACNPs and to nurses who are considering this advanced practice role.

Ellen B. Rudy, PhD, RN, FAAN
Professor and Dean, School of Nursing
University of Pittsburgh

Preface

Acute Care Nurse Practitioners (ACNPs) have entered the arena of advanced practice nursing and have rapidly expanded their roles and practice settings. *Practice Issues for the Acute Care Nurse Practitioner* has been written to provide those practicing and those contemplating practice as an ACNP with resources and information essential to practice. Chapters within the book focus on negotiating and initiating a position as an ACNP, and issues related to practice including collaboration, credentialing, privileging, and evaluation. Additional chapters provide reports from practicing ACNPs in terms of role components and issues affecting practice, and descriptions of ACNP role development in several specialty areas including emergency care and cardiology. Chapter authors are recognized expert ACNP practitioners and educators, and collectively they offer invaluable insight and advice on ACNP practice issues.

Changes in health care will continue to restructure acute care settings and will give rise to new and innovative care delivery settings for ACNP practice. This is an exciting time for ACNPs because they are developing, expanding, and pioneering the role in traditional as well as unique practice settings. Growing numbers of nurses are becoming educated and certified as ACNPs and practice opportunities will continue to expand. *Practice Issues for the Acute Care Nurse Practitioner* provides insight into the developing ACNP role. The book was written as a resource for advanced practice nurses entering or considering roles in advanced practice nursing in acute care. We hope that it will also assist current and future ACNPs to further advance in this exciting new role.

Contributors

Judith G. Baggs, PhD, RN, is an Associate Professor of Nursing and Medical Humanities, University of Rochester School of Nursing

Suzanne M. Burns, MSN, RN, RRT, CCRN, ACNP-CS, is an Associate Professor of Nursing, School of Nursing and Clinician 5–MICU, University of Virginia Health Sciences Center

Janine M. Catalano, MSN, RN, CEN, FNP-C, is a doctoral student in nursing, School of Nursing, and Instructor of Pediatrics, Medical School, the University of Texas Health Science Center at Houston

Frank L. Cole, PhD, RN, CEN, CS, FNP-C, is an Associate Professor of Nursing, Division Head of Emergency Care and Director of Emergency/Ambulatory Care Nurse Practitioner Program at the University of Texas Health Science Center at Houston

Rachel Franklin, MN, RN, CS-ANP, is a Clinical Associate Professor at the University of South Carolina College of Nursing

JoAnne Herman, PhD, RN, is an Associate Professor at the University of South Carolina College of Nursing

Marilyn Hravnak, MSN, RN, ACNP-CS, CCRN, is an Instructor and Manager, Critical Care Subspecialty, Acute Care Nurse Practitioner Program, Acute/Tertiary Care Department, School of Nursing, University of Pittsburgh

Carol Hudgins, MS, RN, ACNP, is an Acute Care Nurse Practitioner, Metro North Cardiovascular Associates, Denton, Texas

Lynn A. Kelso, MSN, ACNP-CS, CCRN, is an Acute Care Nurse Practitioner, MICU, AB Chandler Medical Center and Instructor, University of Kentucky College of Nursing

Kathleen B. King, PhD, RN, is an Associate Professor of Nursing and Psychology, University of Rochester School of Nursing

Marguerite L. Knox, MN, RN, CCRN, CS-ACNP/ANP, is a Clinical Assistant Professor at the University of South Carolina College of Nursing

Kathy Magdic, MSN, RN, CRNP, OCN, is an Instructor and Manager, Cardiopulmonary Subspecialty, Acute Care Nurse Practitioner Program, Acute/Tertiary Care Department, School of Nursing, University of Pittsburgh

Janet S. Nussbaum, EdD, RN, CS-GNP/OCN, is an Assistant Professor at the University of South Carolina College of Nursing

Margaret Q. Rosenzweig, MSN, RN, CRNP-C, AOCN, is a Clinical Instructor, Acute Care Nurse Practitioner Program, Acute/Tertiary Care Department, School of Nursing, University of Pittsburgh

Ellen B. Rudy, PhD, RN, FAAN, is Professor and Dean, School of Nursing, University of Pittsburgh

Deborah Rust, MSN, RN, CRNP, OCN, is an Instructor and Manager, Oncology Subspecialty, Acute Care Nurse Practitioner Program, Acute/ Tertiary Care Department, School of Nursing, University of Pittsburgh

Amelia K. Selph, MN, RN, CS-ACNP, CCRN, is a Clinical Associate Professor at the University of South Carolina College of Nursing

Helen Stupak Shah, DNSc, RN, is an Associate Professor and Interim Associate Dean at the University of Connecticut School of Nursing

Dori Taylor Sullivan, PhD, RN-C, CNA, is Assistant Vice Chancellor, Quality and Performance Improvement, University of Connecticut Health Center

Julie Johnson Zerwic, RN, PhD, is an Assistant Professor at University of Illinois at Chicago College of Nursing

1

Acute Care Nurse Practitioners: Reports From the Practice Setting

Ruth M. Kleinpell

Acute Care Nurse Practitioners (ACNPs) have entered the practice arena of advanced practice nursing and have quickly moved into a variety of practice settings. Although ACNPs continue to work predominantly in tertiary care centers, ACNP roles in secondary and other care facilities have emerged. As of June 1998, there were more than 1200 nurse practitioners who had taken the national ACNP certification exam since it was first offered in December 1995 (American Nurses Credentialing Center, 1998). Surveys from more than 380 of these practitioners reveal that ACNPs are successfully transitioning into various roles with quite an extensive array of responsibilities (Kleinpell, 1997a, 1997b). This chapter will present an overview of practice profiles of ACNPs including issues identified by ACNPs as currently impacting their practice.

THE ROLE OF THE ACUTE CARE NURSE PRACTITIONER

The role of the ACNP was originally developed to fill a need for inpatient care of acutely ill patients. Factors in the formulation of this new category of advanced practice nursing include changes related to managed care and hospital restructuring and changes in medical residency programs, including decreased resident rotation coverage of intensive care units (ICU) and training focus shift to primary care (Daly & Genet, 1997; Ingersoll, 1995; Keane, Richmond, & Kaiser, 1994; Kindig & Libby, 1994; Parrinello, 1995).

Although some of the first ACNP practitioners were adult nurse practitioners or tertiary nurse practitioners trained specifically for certain roles in inpatient settings, graduate degree ACNP programs began to emerge in the late 1980s and rapidly flourished. Currently, there are more than 70 educational programs that offer ACNP education at the master's or post master's level (American Association of Colleges of Nursing, 1998; American Association of Critical Care Nurses, 1996).

The publication of the *Standards of Clinical Practice and Scope of Practice for the Acute Care Nurse Practitioner* (American Nurses Association, 1995) and the availability of a national certification for ACNPs can be viewed as the "official" recognition of the ACNP as a new category of advanced practice nursing. Positions for ACNPs have emerged predominantly in ICU and acute care areas within the hospital setting. In the early days, the ACNP often functioned in physician extender roles that closely paralleled the work of residents or house staff physicians. Other ACNPs were pioneers in practice arenas where an advanced practitioner was needed to directly manage patient care.

As the holistic care aspects of the nurse practitioner role became evident in practice, ACNP roles emerged that combined aspects of medical and nursing care management of patients in a variety of practice settings. ACNPs report practicing in many areas, including hospital-based ICU settings, emergency rooms, trauma care, and specialty-based practice in oncology, transplantation, neurology, and multipractice clinic sites (Gaedeke & Blount, 1995; Gedwill, Mack, Mlakar, & Vanek, 1997; Genet et al., 1995; Giacalone, Mullaney, DeJoseph, & Cosma, 1995; Kelso & Massaro, 1994; Kleinpell, 1997a, 1997b; Martin & Coniglio, 1996). Expansion of the role to subacute care, rehabilitation, home care, interventional radiology, and other areas has also occurred. Table 1.1 outlines practice specialty areas reported by practicing ACNPs.

As the practice settings for ACNPs have expanded, so too have components of the role. ACNPs are no longer viewed as merely physician extenders. ACNP roles consist of conducting histories and physical exams, planning patient care, monitoring lab and test results, performing procedures, and initiating consults, transfers, and discharges. Although ACNPs

TABLE 1.1 Specialty Practice Areas of ACNPs

Cardiothoracic ICU	Surgical ICU	Coronary ICU	Medical ICU
Medical rehabilitation	Neurology ICU	Multipractice clinic	Trauma
Stepdown unit/telemetry	Catheterization lab	Subacute care	Emergency
Infectious disease clinic	Craniofacial surgery	Endocrinology	Home care
Interventional cardiology	Internal medicine	Urgent care center	Transplant
Rheumatology clinic	Diabetic clinic	Pulmonary medicine	Nephrology
ENT/Plastic surgery group	Orthopaedics	Oncology	Radiology
Medical flight program	Gerontology	Employee health	
Mental health services	Presurgical testing	Private practice MD	

report performing a variety of patient care procedures, the most frequently cited responsibilities include ordering and interpreting laboratory tests and x-rays; interpreting 12–lead electrocardiograms; managing medication, oxygenation, fluid, and nutrition therapies; pain management; and discussing care with family members. Performing specialty procedures such as wound debridement and suturing, thoracentesis, bone marrow aspiration, inserting invasive monitoring catheters, intubation, or resuscitation management often depends on the practice specialty area of the ACNP.

A common misperception is that ACNPs are performing extensive and invasive procedural work that traditionally was within a physician's scope of practice. ACNP educational programs do not routinely teach invasive skill acquisition, and often the ACNP gains exposure to performing procedures when employed in a role managing specific patient populations, for example, cardiology, neurology, or oncology patients. Although performing patient care procedures can be part of the role, ACNPs report that overseeing, managing, and providing care consistency are major aspects of their role. Other role components can include teaching (nursing staff, patients and family members, medical and nurse practitioner students), research, program development, department projects, quality assurance work, and committee participation.

To demonstrate how ACNP practice and role components are in part determined by the practice setting, the following sections outline several ACNP roles in different practice settings.

The Long-Term Acute Care Setting

An ACNP working in a long-term acute care setting for patients who require wound care, ventilator weaning, rehabilitation, or continued treatment of complex medical problems after hospitalization reports that she directly manages patients in collaboration with private practice physicians. In this setting, two ACNPs provide Monday through Friday coverage of service patients. Job components include daily patient rounds, ordering and interpreting diagnostic and laboratory tests, adjusting or changing medications, and managing medical problems in conjunction with the service physician. In addition, interactions with the patient's family and interdisciplinary team members, including representatives from physical therapy, occupational therapy, respiratory therapy, dietetics and psychiatry, and planning for discharge needs make the ACNP role a truly comprehensive one in this type of setting.

The Neurosurgical Intensive Care Unit

A unit-based ACNP in a neurosurgical ICU reports that major role components include daily follow through on patient progress and performing detailed neurological examinations. It is important to detect subtle changes in level of consciousness and functional abilities in neurosurgical patients. Because nursing staff and resident physicians often rotate patient assignments, the role of the ACNP in monitoring the ongoing neurological status of the patient becomes an integral component of patient management. Following protocols, the ACNP independently orders indicated treatments and performs such procedures as inserting and managing lumbar and extraventricular drains, performs lumbar punctures, and oversees intracranial monitoring. Currently, this ACNP is also involved in staff nurse education and in data collection for a research project exploring risk factors for the development of vasospasm in patients with aneuryms.

The Urology Service

An ACNP working for an inpatient urology service identified that the role entails assessment and follow-up of all inpatient and outpatient clinic patients referred to the service. Primary responsibilities include taking a history and conducting physical exams, ordering and interpreting laboratory and diagnostic tests, and initiating indicated treatments. Other role responsibilities include assisting in the operating room, teaching, and inservice education to staff nurses and residents. Procedures performed by the ACNP include straight catheterizations for urinary retention, suprapubic needle aspirations, bladder irrigation, bladder scans, and interpretation of intravenous pyelograms, cystograms, and other ultrasonography tests.

Patients often present with a variety of urologic conditions, including hematuria, obstructive uropathies, urinary tract infections, hydronephrosis, renal failure, stress incontinence, calculi, and prostatitis. Therefore, the ability to efficiently and accurately diagnose and manage patient's urologic conditions is essential to this ACNP's role.

The Bone Marrow Transplant Program

An ACNP employed in a bone marrow transplant program reports being responsible for both inpatients and outpatients. In the inpatient setting, the ACNP sees and examines patients independently and formulates a preliminary plan of care, including ordering and evaluating laboratory and radiological tests. A collaborative plan is then made based on consultation with the attending physician team. The ACNP follows patients until hospital discharge, making daily changes to the plan of care based on patient progress and assessment data. The ACNP is responsible for managing a caseload of patients and independently consulting others, such as cardiology, pulmonary medicine, dermatology, or infectious disease specialists to manage concurrent patient conditions. In the outpatient setting, the ACNP performs the initial physical examination, orders indicated tests, and prescribes treatment changes and medications in consultation with the attending physician. Biweekly on-call time is also included in the ACNP's role responsibilities.

The Emergency Room Setting

An ACNP working in an emergency room setting rotates between a fast track area and an observation unit within the emergency room. The ACNP independently examines and assesses the patient, performs indicated testing, and consults with the emergency room physician on the appropriate treatment. In the fast track area, the ACNP often evaluates patients who present with fractures, sprains, eye injuries, low back pain, pharyngitis, and lacerations. Procedure work may include wound irrigations and debridement, suturing, nerve blocks, joint aspirations and reductions, and use of a slit lamp to check for corneal abrasions.

Other patients require a more in-depth workup for conditions such as abdominal pain or dehydration. The ACNP may need to admit these patients to the general emergency room and monitor the patient for an extended period of time. In addition to assessment and treatment of a variety of patient conditions, patient education is also a major component of this ACNP's position.

The Subacute Geriatric Setting

An ACNP on a subacute skilled geriatric unit reports that role components include going on daily patient rounds; managing acute issues such as changes in vital signs, confusion, and wound care assessment and management; evaluating patient responses to treatment and medications; and subsequently changing the treatment plan in consultation with the attending physician. Additional role responsibilities include coordinating interdisciplinary team meetings for discharge planning issues, staff nurse education, skill validation for such procedures as port-a-cath management, and serving as a resource consultant for other geriatric units in the facility on such issues as central line care, splinting, and proper patient positioning. Because many of the patients have complex discharge needs, the ACNP also works closely with family members in evaluating home care or secondary placement issues.

The Cardiology Service

An ACNP working on an inpatient cardiology service reports that role responsibilities include admitting patients, taking histories and conducting physical exams, ordering indicated tests and treatments based on protocol orders, and interpreting laboratory and diagnostic tests. Other aspects of the role include initiating needed consults, such as with the pulmonary or renal department, and conferring with the cardiology team regarding the indicated plan of care. Additional responsibilities include patient and family teaching in terms of medications and procedures such as angiograms, stress tests, coronary artery bypass graft surgery; overseeing and coordinating discharge planning; and making community service referrals.

The Community Health Clinic Setting

An ACNP working in a rural community health center reports that the role is family practice–based and includes seeing clinic patients, treating acute and emergent care conditions, and taking call at a nearby 40-bed hospital to cover service patients. Although practice in the clinic is autonomous, hospital practice is governed by protocols and care is required to be sponsored and supervised by a physician. Additional role components include initiating patient consults and transfers to other service facilities and hospital committee work.

PRACTICE ISSUES OF ACUTE CARE NURSE PRACTITIONERS

In addition to describing aspects of their practice, ACNPs identified issues having an impact on their practice, including role recognition and acceptance and ability to use all their skills. One ACNP related, "Many with whom I work are not quite sure what to expect in this role. We don't fit into any specific category—we are not a staff nurse, not a physician, not a physician's assistant, not a "family" nurse practitioner. We are really carving out our role" (Kleinpell, 1997b). Another commented, "Many persons do not understand the role of the ACNP. In order to utilize the ACNP to the fullest potential, an adequate understanding of the role is necessary" (Kleinpell, 1997b).

Some ACNPs have experienced resistence to the role from physicians and nursing colleagues. One ACNP commented "It has been challenging to educate physicians on ACNP definition and utilization. It has been challenging to implement a new role in the hospital in terms of job description, salary, practice guidelines and privileges" (Kleinpell, 1997b). Another comment was "I never imagined the resistance to my role from other nurses. Is it jealousy? Some doctors won't talk to me and some secretaries won't put me through to the doctor for a direct call" (Kleinpell, 1997b). Another ACNP commented, "There are now only two ACNPs where I work. We anticipate that nursing may be the most difficult one to accept the role. This stems from how invisible nursing has usually been to itself and others. Even though one can describe, show, define what a nurse is and does, you so often sense that others do not attribute the same to the nurse" (Kleinpell, 1997b).

Transitioning into the ACNP role can be challenging but rewarding. One ACNP related, "This is a new position that continues to evolve. I believe this to be a unique opportunity, one full of autonomy and tremendous avenues to impact change" (Kleinpell, 1997b).

SUMMARY

The practice components of these ACNPs reveal that the role of the ACNP can be truly multifaceted. Common elements of the ACNP role exist regardless of the practice setting or specialty area, such as performing history and physical exams, ordering and interpreting laboratory and diagnostic tests, directly managing patient care in collaboration with the physician, and evaluating responses to treatment. Other role components such as performing procedures and diagnostic test interpretation and evaluation depend on the type of patients seen by the ACNP.

ACNPs are currently practicing in a tremendous variety of roles. The areas in which ACNPs can effect change in order to render improved collaborative care remain broad based and extensive. As health-care changes continue to occur, movement of ACNPs to acute care outpatient settings, worksite clinics, and other innovative practice areas to meet market needs will occur. As new practice settings evolve for the ACNP, role components will also continue to expand.

REFERENCES

American Association of Colleges of Nursing. (1998). *Peterson's guide to nursing programs: Baccalaureate and graduate nursing education in the U.S. and Canada.* Princeton, NJ: Peterson's Guides, Inc.

American Association of Critical Care Nurses. (1996). *Graduate Nursing Programs.* Aliso Viejo, CA: Author.

American Nurses Association. (1995). *Standards of clinical practice and scope of practice for the acute care nurse practitioner.* Washington, DC: American Nurses Publishing.

American Nurses Credentialing Center. (1998). Washington, DC.

Daly, B., & Genet, C. (1997). Influence of the health care environment. In B. Daly (Ed.), *The acute care nurse practitioner* (pp. 29–56). New York: Springer Publishing.

Gaedeke, M., & Blount, K. (1995). Advanced practice nursing in pediatric acute care. *Critical Care Nursing Clinics of North America, 1,* 61–70.

Gedwill, A., Mack, S., Mlakar, D., & Vanek, R. (1997). Actualization of the ACNP role: The experience of university hospitals of Cleveland. In B. Daly (Ed.), *The acute care nurse practitioner* (pp. 141–170). New York: Springer Publishing.

Genet, C., Brennan, P., Ibbotson-Wolff, S., et al. (1995). Nurse practitioners in a teaching hospital. *Nurse Practitioner, 9,* 47–54.

Giacalone, M., Mullaney, D., DeJoseph, D., Cosma, M. (1995). Development of a nurse-managed unit and the advanced practitioner role. *Critical Care Clinics of North America, 1,* 35–41.

Ingersoll, G. (1995). Evaluation of the advanced practice nurse role in acute and specialty care. *Critical Care Nursing Clinics of North America, 7,* 25–34.

Keane, A., Richmond, T., & Kaiser, L. (1994). Critical care nurse practitioners: Evolution of the advanced practice nursing role. *American Journal of Critical Care, 3,* 232–237.

Kelso, L., & Massaro, L. (1994). Implementation of the acute care nurse practitioner role. *AACN Clinical Issues, 3,* 404–407.

Kingid, D., & Libby, D. (1994). How will graduate medical education reform affect specialties and geographic areas? *Journal of the American Medical Association, 1,* 37–42.

Kleinpell, R. (1997a). Acute-care nurse practitioners: roles and practice profiles. *AACN Clinical Issues, 8,* 156–162.

Kleinpell, R. (1997b). Survey of acute care nurse practitioners. Paper presented at the Fifth Annual Acute Care Nurse Practitioner Consensus Conference, April 19, Myrtle Beach, South Carolina.

Martin, B., & Coniglio, J. (1996). The acute care nurse practitioner in collaborative practice. *AACN Clinical Issues, 2,* 309–314.

Parrinello, K. (1995). Advanced practice nursing. *Critical Care Nursing Clinics of North America, 1,* 9–16.

2

Demonstrating the Effectiveness of Acute Care Nurse Practitioners: Current and Future Research

Mariann R. Piano and Julie Johnson Zerwic

In tertiary care settings, the profession of nursing has seen an emergence of the acute care nurse practitioner (ACNP). Although the first practicing ACNP dates back to 1960, it has only been within the last few years that the popularity and demand for the ACNP has occurred within tertiary care settings (McGivern, 1993). To date, there are more than 50 nursing graduate programs with an ACNP program option (American Association of Colleges of Nursing [AACN], 1995). Since this is a new role it is important to document ACNP-directed positive health care outcomes. The purpose of this chapter is to review the literature for evidence of ACNP effectiveness in the acute care setting, in terms of short-and long-term patient outcomes. In addition, this chapter will provide recommendations for future ACNP outcomes research. Prior to reviewing the ACNP patient outcome literature, the definition of an ACNP is provided, along with a brief overview of ACNP educational preparation.

TERMS AND DEFINITION OF AN ACUTE CARE NURSE PRACTITIONER

The term tertiary nurse practitioner was initially used by the nursing profession and appeared in the literature to denote an advanced practice nurse working in an acute or tertiary care setting. The term tertiary was used initially to emphasize the difference in practice settings between the ACNP and other advanced practice nurses and nurse practitioners (NPs) who provided care in primary care settings. Others have also referred to the acute care advanced practice nurse according to her or his practice or speciality setting, for example, trauma nurse practitioners, pediatric nurse practitioners, and critical care nurse practitioners. In the literature over the last few years, however, the term ACNP is most often used when referring to advanced practice nurses in acute care settings. In this chapter the acute care advanced practice nurse will be referred to as an ACNP.

The ACNP is defined as an advanced practice nurse who is engaged primarily in providing care to complex, acutely ill patients. In most situations the patients have multiple acute and chronic health problems (Piano, Kleinpell, & Johnson, 1996). Similar to other advanced practice nurses, ACNPs are required to assess patients, think critically, perform diagnostic reasoning, manage cases, and prescribe therapeutic interventions (Clochesy, Daley, Idemoto, Steel, & Fitzpatrick, 1993; Keane & Richmond, 1993).

EDUCATIONAL BACKGROUND FOR ACUTE CARE NURSE PRACTITIONERS

ACNPs are prepared with 2 to 3 years of graduate education. The educational curriculum is quite rigorous and includes advanced courses in pharmacology, physiology, health assessment, and patient management. In most states, ACNPs are baccalaureate-prepared licensed registered nurses who have completed a graduate program in nursing and obtained a master's degree. ACNP educational curriculum is based on the educational or curricular standards for *Clinical Practice and Scope of Practice for the Acute Care Nurse Practitioner* (AACN, 1995).

The curriculum includes a master's core, an advanced practice core, and a specialty theory or clinical core. The master's core consists of research, statistics, and nursing theory courses; the advanced practice core comprises advanced physiology, pathophysiology, pharmacology, and health assessment classes. Depending on the ACNP's area of specialization (i.e., cardiopulmonary, critical care, oncology), the ACNP completes a series of specialty-related pathophysiology and management classes and clinical practicums. Finally, prior to entering the ACNP program most of the ACNPs have an average of 5 years of nursing experience in their specialty area.

Considering the preceding, it appears that ACNPs are well prepared to provide care within their specialty area. Education aside, it remains important to demonstrate that ACNP practice is evidence based and care outcomes are similar to those of physicians and other health-care professionals.

REVIEW OF OUTCOME STUDIES ON ACUTE CARE NURSE PRACTITIONERS

The effectiveness of NPs in health care settings has been debated since the inception of the role in the late 1960's (Buppert Knight, 1995). More than 200 studies have been conducted to examine NP effectiveness. Brown and Grimes (1995) have provided a summary of these reports and meta-analysis of primary NP and midwife patient care outcomes. Reports in this chapter were therefore limited to those involving ACNPs in tertiary care settings.

Manual and computerized MEDLINE searches were conducted using the following key terms: nurse practitioner, acute care nurse practitioner, tertiary nurse practitioner, and patient outcomes and effectiveness. Using multiple combinations of these key terms, more than 150 articles were identified. Articles ranged from descriptions of ACNP questionnaire tools to NP-directed case management protocols; however, few articles were research studies. Brown and Grimes (1995) identified several criteria that they used to select studies for their meta-analysis on NP effectiveness. For example, three of the six criteria were as follows: "(1) an intervention provided by an NP/nurse midwife (NM) or NP-physician/NM-physician team, (2) an experimental, quasi-experimental or ex post facto research design, and (3) data that permitted calculation of effect sizes and/or determination of direction of effects" (Brown & Grimes, 1995, p. 34). Using these criteria, however, there were not sufficient data to conduct a meta-analysis on ACNP effectiveness. Therefore, in selecting ACNP studies the following guidelines were used to identify relevant studies: advanced practice nurse responsible for patient management, tertiary care setting, measurement of some type of patient-related outcome and comparisons made between the ACNP and other types of health-care professionals. Using these guidelines, only eight studies were identified, and in some reports the care provided by an ACNP and another health care professional (physician assistant [PA]) were studied together (e.g., NP/PA care compared with physician care). A summary of the research conducted thus far in this field is presented in Table 2.1 and includes prospective as well as descriptive (qualitative) studies of the ACNP role.

Very few of the reports in Table 2.1 met the rigorous research standards set by the scientific community; however, this summary will provide new insights for developing ACNP outcome research. Most of the studies summarized in Table 2.1 were associated with positive health care outcomes. For example, Spisso, O'Callaghan, McKennan, & Holcroft (1990) found that the addition of ACNPs to the trauma team had a marked impact on such outcomes as patient compliance with outpatient follow-up, patient length of stay, and patient complaints. Mitchell-DiCenso et al. (1996) and Carzoli, Martinez-Cruz, Cuevas, & Murphy (1994) found that the NP or clinical nurse specialist (CNS) in conjunction with PAs delivered care comparable to that provided by attending physicians and physicians in training. Although the sample size was small, the findings of Cintron, Bigas, Linates, Aranda, and Hernandez (1983) and Ziemer et al. (1996) suggest that in special patient populations, such as heart failure and diabetes patients, respectively, the impact of NP-directed clinics is associated with a favorable effect on patient outcomes. This is not surprising since these types of patients may require more follow-up and monitoring. Collectively, it appears that in the tertiary care setting, NP-directed patient outcomes were similar to their respective comparison group and NP-directed care was cost effective.

The studies in Table 2.1 demonstrate ACNP effectiveness in several types of tertiary care settings. The findings must be interpreted with caution, however, due to methodological flaws that include lack of randomization and appropriate control or comparison groups and insufficient sample size. The majority of these reports were retrospective and used historical data (Carzoli et al., 1994; Cintron et al., 1983; Hooker & McCaig, 1996; Lombness, 1994; Spisso et al., 1990; Weinberg, Lijestrand, & Moore, 1983). Several of these studies included a cost analysis; however, it was not always clear how the costs were calculated and which costs were considered (i.e., house staff salaries, work hours, total col-

TABLE 2.1 Summary of ACNP Studies

Study Citation	Type of ACNP/Educational Preparation	Study Design	Setting/Comparison Group	Outcome Measures and Findings
Spisso J, et al. (1990)	Trauma ACNP/RNs with previous surgical intensive care/acute care experience Indicated that trauma ACNPs completed an NP program	Retrospective study design comparing numerous outcomes pre-and post-NP implementation in a trauma outpatient setting	Trauma outpatient setting No comparison group; investigators collectively evaluated the overall impact of ACNPs on the trauma team's outcomes	Classified outcome measures into two groups: cost benefits and impact on health care team *Findings*: ↑ compliance with outpatient follow-up exams; ↑ nursing staff and house staff satisfaction with ACNP role; ↑ follow-up referral; ↑ compliance with review of systems; ↓ patient length of stay (LOS); ↓ outpatient waiting times; ↓ patient complaints
Mitchell-DiCenso et al. (1996)	CNS/NP RNs (Separate designation between CNS and NP was not made) CNS/NP educated in a 16-month graduate NP program	Prospective, randomized controlled study Neonates were randomly assigned to receive care by the CNS/NP team or neonatal intensive care unit (NICU) staff	NICU NICU staff: neonatologist, neonatal fellow, residents	Outcomes measured: mortality, number of neonatal complications, LOS, quality of care, parent satisfaction, long-term outcomes, medical and family costs *Findings:* There were no significant differences between any of the above outcomes measured between CNS/NP and the neonatal staff
Hooker & McCaig (1996)	The type of NP designated was described as NP	Retrospective (exploratory) study design, which	ED Physician/clinic group	This report was primarily an exploratory (survey) study

TABLE 2.1 *Continued*

Study Citation	Type of ACNP/Educational Preparation	Study Design	Setting/Comparison Group	Outcome Measures and Findings
	employed in an emergency department (ED) setting NPs were grouped with PAs and designated as the NP/PA group	analyzed data from the National Ambulatory Medical Care Survey		designed to examine use of NP/PA in ED settings, types of ED patients seen by NP/PAs, drugs prescribed by NP/PAs, diagnostic screening services and actual diagnosis made by NP/PAs *Findings:* There were no clinically significant differences in the above variables between the NP/PA group and other physicians/clinic groups
Ziemer et al. (1996)	NPs and RNs (RNs had speciality education in diabetes) NP educational preparation was not noted	Prospective study of patients with diabetes (type II) over a 12–month period	Diabetes unit in a hospital setting No control group	Outcomes studied were disease specific and included glycemic control (blood glucose level), diet and weight control, metabolic control (hemoglobin A1c levels) *Findings:* All outcomes were markedly improved, and these outcomes were achieved primarily through improved nonpharmacologic therapies such as diet control and weight loss

Continued

TABLE 2.1 *Continued*

Study Citation	Type of ACNP/Educational Preparation	Study Design	Setting/Comparison Group	Outcome Measures and Findings
Carzoli et al. (1994)	Neonatal nurse practitioners (NNP) NNP education included completion of a 9-month certificate NP program NPs were grouped with PAs and referred to as the PA/NP group	Retrospective chart review (6-month study period)	NICU Residents in training	Outcomes included NICU and total LOS, total parental nutrition use, number of blood transfusions, performance on various procedures, complications (i.e., incidence of air leaks, bronchopulmonary dysplasia etc.) and infant mortality. *Findings*: There were no differences in NICU or total LOS; similarly there were no differences in any other outcomes between groups including mortality. When comparing annual costs (including services and salaries) and hospital charges, however, NP/PA care was associated with an overall cost savings
Cintron et al. (1983)	NP Detail regarding NP education not included	Retrospective chart review	NP heart failure (HF) clinic	Outcomes for 15 HF patients were studied and included total number of hospitalizations, number of hospitalized days,

TABLE 2.1 *Continued*

Study Citation	Type of ACNP/Educational Preparation	Study Design	Setting/Comparison Group	Outcome Measures and Findings
				and total medical costs. These outcomes were evaluated before and after the implementation of the HF clinic *Findings*: After implementation of the clinic there was a 60% reduction in number of hospitalizations and an 85% reduction in the mean number of hospitalized days. Medical costs were also markedly reduced. Because of the small sample size, however, these findings may not be generalizable to other HF patients.
Weinberg et al. (1983)	NP Educated in a hospital-affiliated NP program	Retrospective chart review	Stroke rehabilitation unit Physician internists	The following outcomes were evaluated over a 6-month period in 25 stroke patients: LOS, laboratory and x-ray costs per day, number of consultations and management of common medical problems (e.g., urinary tract infection, congestive heart failure, diabetes, etc.).

Continued

TABLE 2.1 *Continued*

Study Citation	Type of ACNP/Educational Preparation	Study Design	Setting/Comparison Group	Outcome Measures and Findings
				Findings: No differences were found between patients assigned to the NP unit or independent internist unit
Lombness (1994)	CNS Master's degree in nursing	Descriptive, retrospective chart review.	Cardiovascular (CV) surgery unit PAs	Outcomes measured included ICU-LOS, ICU + step-down LOS and CV-related complications *Findings*: These investigators found that LOS (ICU and ICU + step-down) was shorter in the CNS-managed group compared with patients in the PA managed group, whereas there were no differences in the overall incidence of complications

In most of the above reports, the nurse practitioners were designated according to their practice setting (e.g., trauma nurse practitioner, neonatal nurse practitioner). Therefore the acronym ACNP was not used in the above table. Abbreviations used: PA-physicians assistant, ED-Emergency Department, ER-emergency room, NP-nurse practitioner, RN-registered nurse, CNS-Clinical Nurse specialist.

lected fees, etc.) (Carzoli et al., 1994; Cintron et al., 1983; Mitchell-DiCenso et al., 1996; Weinberg et al., 1983). As discussed later, future studies need to be developed that are multisite and prospective and incorporate a control comparison group.

DEVELOPMENT OF STUDIES TO EXAMINE ACUTE CARE NURSE PRACTITIONER OUTCOMES

In order to document the effectiveness of the ACNP role, well-designed studies must be conducted. For several decades researchers have examined the more established advance practice roles such as NM and primary care NP. Although there are a substantial number of studies, convincing evidence to support these roles has been limited. This is because the studies have lacked acceptable conceptual definitions and measurement of variables and have not used the appropriate methodological controls necessary to provide valid conclusions (Brown & Grimes, 1995). In order to provide support for the validity of the ACNP role, the lessons learned from the earlier advanced nursing practice literature must be examined.

Measures of Acute Care Nurse Practitioner Effectiveness in Health Care

Measures of the ACNP effectiveness can be organized into the following categories: the processes of health care, the outcomes of health care, patients' satisfaction with care, and agreement between NP and physician decisions (Sox, 1979). The process category includes variables dealing with the type or amount of care delivered (Prescott & Driscoll, 1979). For example, process variables could include procedures or tests such as the number of x-rays ordered and relevant data obtained and documented during a history and physical examination. Most studies have used process variables that focused on the medical or cure components of health care (Prescott & Driscoll, 1979). Obviously, if the public is interested in identifying whether an NP can assume some of the responsibilities typically designated as medical, the focus of evaluation will be on the aspects of the NP role that focus on cure. It is important, however, that these variables not be the sole measures of the effectiveness of the role. For example, patients who receive care provided by ACNPs may have an improved quality of life that is a result of the counseling or education activities associated with the nursing component of the ACNP role.

Outcome of health care refers to the short- and long-term outcomes of health care delivery. Examples of short-term outcomes could include measures that relate to specific diseases and therapies, such as blood pressure normalization in hypertensive patients or glycemic control in diabetes patients. Other short-term measures that are more general include hospital length of stay, physical functioning, readmission, and mortality. Another important outcome variable is a cost analysis that incorporates provider costs (salaries and hours worked per week) and cost associated with procedures and hospitalization. When analyzing ACNP effectiveness, long-term as well as short-term outcomes should be included. In a review by Crosby, Ventura, and Feldman (1987), however, only 14% of 248 studies used long-term outcomes. Both short- and long-term outcome measures reflect the goal of health care and therefore both types should be used. Finally, even though some of the outcome measures can be directly attributable to specific provider interventions and therapies, other short-and long-term outcomes are beyond the control of the caregiver. For example, patient variables, such as income, education, and available support systems, which can significantly influence outcomes, are beyond the control of all health care providers (Sox, 1979).

Patient satisfaction can be assessed directly by asking patients' to share their feelings about the care they received or may be observed indirectly by examining patient compliance with follow-up visits. Patient satisfaction is an important variable to assess because it is a reflection of the acceptance of NPs. Patient satisfaction, however, does not necessarily equate with quality of care and thus should never be the sole variable in a study of NP effectiveness.

Agreement between NPs and physicians has been used as an outcome variable in studies in which both practitioners independently examined the same patient and their decisions were compared (Sox, 1979). This method is infrequently used because only the process of care can be studied; it is impossible to identify which practitioner had the greatest impact on outcome. In addition, it is expensive to have multiple practitioners seeing the same patient, and the patient may interact with providers differently depending on what happened during the first provider interaction.

There are limited data delineating external criteria against which NP performance can be judged; therefore, NP performance is compared with the extent to which the NP practices like a physician. For example, in the assessment of a patient the NP would be expected to identify the same problems that a physician had and order the same diagnostic tests.

This presents a difficulty because the NP can never exceed the performance of a physician. There are a few studies in which a specific standard of care was identified and then the performance of all practitioners was compared to that standard (Avron, Everitt, & Baker, 1991). This type of comparison may be more equitable for ACNPs.

To date, based on the recent literature, it appears there is no difference between ACNPs and other health care providers (Hooker & McCaig, 1996; Mitchell-DiCenso et al., 1996; Weinberg et al., 1983). These findings may have been a result of selecting variables that were not sensitive enough to detect significant differences between groups. Careful attention should be given to the choice of the measurement outcomes (Prescott & Driscoll, 1979). Measurement outcomes that are specific to a particular situation or health problem may be more sensitive than are global measures. This sensitivity may be necessary to detect differences and increase the credibility of the findings. This does present a threat to the generalizability of the results, however, because the findings from very specific measures may only be generalized to clients with similar conditions. In addition, it is important that outcome variables are selected that realistically can be influenced by ACNP management.

Methodological Design Considerations

There are a number of methodological issues that should be considered before initiating a study in order to provide valid results. Although it may not be possible to implement a study under ideal conditions, a number of safeguards or controls can be built into the study in order to provide realistic comparisons between groups. In addition, information that should be provided in all published studies will be described. Certain information should be available to the readers to enhance generalizing the results as well as facilitating future meta-analysis of NP studies. The remainder of this chapter outlines issues in study design that should be recognized prior to study development.

Provider Sample and Setting

The health care providers who are to be compared should be chosen carefully. Often the provider(s) include a small number of individuals chosen because of convenience. The more providers included, the more likely it will be that the conclusions can be generalized to other providers. Random sampling of providers is the preferred method of selection. If this cannot be done, then careful selection of practitioners to represent variability in terms of experience and length of time in practice is acceptable (Prescott & Driscoll, 1979).

The comparison group for ACNPs should be considered carefully. NPs could be compared with residents with little experience or physicians who are likely to have more experience. The comparison will likely depend on the purpose of the study. If the goal is to document that ACNPs can assume responsibilities that had been assigned to a resident group, then residents should be the likely comparison group. Other groups, such as PAs, might serve as a comparison group.

The characteristics of all providers, both NPs and comparison health care providers, should be identified explicitly. NP education and training has not been standardized. Only recently has NP education required a master's degree. In addition, practitioners can vary widely in their experience and years of practice. Researchers also need to consider the clinical experience of the ACNP. For example, prior to entering the ACNP master's program, some ACNP may have more than 12 years in a specific area, such as critical care or trauma nursing.

A complete description of the practice environment must be provided. For example, findings from a study conducted in a closed ICU directed by a medical intensivist may be very different from the results from an open ICU where attendings are ultimately responsible for patient care decisions. A careful and detailed description will facilitate the ability to generalize the results of the study.

Patient Sample

The sample size needs to be carefully considered. Including too few patients can limit the ability to detect differences between the groups. A power analysis can provide information about the sample size that is needed based on the outcome variables that will be used.

A detailed description of the patient sample is critical to the generalizability of the results. In the past, studies have been criticized because patients who received care from NPs were believed to have a lower acuity than patients cared for by the comparison group (Brown & Grimes, 1995). An appropriate study design should control for differences in patient acuity; however, it is important to provide data about patient demographics, pretreatment status, and severity of current health problems in order to ensure equivalence across groups. Information about patients who drop out of the study should also be provided.

Design

One of the major criticisms of the research on NP effectiveness is the lack of rigor in the research design. Random assignment of patients to providers is necessary to control for patient morbidity (Brown & Grimes, 1995). Random allocation of patients ensures equitable distribution of all sources of bias to both the experimental and the control groups (Sox, 1979).

The data collection should occur concurrently for both groups in the same or equivalent practice settings. Often, studies are designed in which the data are collected from NPs during one time period and the comparison group during another time period. It is possible that the results could be confounded by events occurring during one time period that were unrelated to the study.

Multiple data sources and multiple outcomes should be used (Sox, 1979). The use of several data sources and measurement of more than one outcome would help to identify both the scope and the limitations of NP practice. In addition, the attention of the investigation should be on the *system of care* rather than on the practitioner (Brown & Grimes, 1995). Providing detailed information in published reports about the care activities of the different practitioners will facilitate relating specific activities to care outcomes. Finally, to facilitate the comparison of results across studies, summary statistics must be published.

Carefully consider the research team that is developed. It is important that the results be viewed as credible and free of bias. In order to ensure that the data are recognized as reliable and valid it may be necessary to include individuals from different perspectives (e.g., physicians) and individuals who do not have a stake in the outcome of the study.

SUMMARY

In tertiary care settings, the ACNP has become an important addition to the health care team. Even though to date there are insufficient data to support their role, it is anticipated that ACNPs will have a marked impact on the delivery of health care. For example, unlike residents, ACNPs are a consistent member of the health care team. Therefore, they are able to maintain the continuity of patient care during frequent resident transitions or rotations. In addition, health care has become highly technical, requiring expertise in specialized areas such as hemodynamic

TABLE 2.2 Health-Related Outcome Measures

Patient health knowledge	Mortality
Patient compliance	Nursing staff turnover and retention
Health maintenance	Interdisciplinary patient planning
Return for follow-up	Unit residency hours and shift rotation
Number of inpatient days	Complications
Office visits	Number of procedures (invasive and noninvasive)
Health care utilization	Quality of life
Relationship between the setting characteristics and specific patient outcomes	Functional status
Recividism	Patient satisfaction
Employee satisfaction	Infection rates
Symptom management and symptom control	

monitoring and respiratory therapy. ACNPs that have completed practicums in specialized areas, such as critical care, can provide the health care team with this expertise. An ACNP's education also includes the principles of patient education, family dynamics, and health maintenance. Therefore, it is not unlikely that the ACNP would have an impact on such outcomes as patient health knowledge, patient compliance, health maintenance, and health care use. These important outcomes need to be included and measured in ACNP studies.

Measured outcome variables need to be specific to the population of interest and the appropriate care setting. The most commonly used outcome variables are endpoints such as mortality and morbidity and the cost savings. Other outcome variables, however, are listed in Table 2.2 and are important to consider and should be incorporated into a research study. There is also a prevailing notion that ACNP practice is not supported by physician and resident colleagues. Yet there is not a substantial amount of data to support this notion. In fact, Spisso et al. (1990) reported that other trauma health care team members (such as attending physicians and residents) had very favorable attitudes toward the ACNP.

In conclusion, it will be important to demonstrate that ACNP practice is associated with positive health care outcomes and to address the following four questions stated by Oakland and Followell (1990, p. 13): "Can we do the job correctly? (capability) Are we doing the job correctly? (control) Have we done the job correctly? (quality assurance) Could we do the job better? (improvement)"

For centuries, other types of industry have systematically studied the process of quality control and outcome by addressing the four questions above. Only recently, however, have health care professionals been challenged to address these same questions. Although it will be an arduous task, it is important that in answering the above questions, ACNPs collect data prospectively using a randomized study design and appropriate control or comparison groups.

REFERENCES

American Association of Colleges of Nursing. (1995). *The Essentials of Master's Education for Advanced Practice Nursing.* Washington, DC: Author.

American Nurses Association. (1995). Standards for Clinical Practice and Scope of Practice for the Acute Care Nurse Practitioner. Washington, DC: Author.

Avron, J., Everitt, D.E., & Baker, M.W. (1991). The neglected medical history and therapeutic choices for abdominal pain: A nationwide study of 799 physicians and nurses. *Archives of Internal Medicine, 151,* 694–698.

Brown, S. A., & Grimes, D.E. (1995). A meta-analysis of nurse practitioners and nurse midwives in primary care. *Nursing Research, 44*(6), 332–339.

Buppert Knight, C. (1995). Justifying nurse practitioner existence: Hard facts to hard figures. *Nurse Practitioner, 20*(8), 43–48.

Carzoli, R.P., Martinez-Cruz, M., Cuevas, L.L., & Murphy, S. (1994). Comparison of neonatal practitioners, physician assistants, and residents in the neonatal intensive care unit. *Archives of Pediatric Adolescence, 148,* 1271–1276.

Cintron, G., Bigas, C., Linates, E., Aranda, J.M., & Hernandez, E. (1983). Nurse practitioner role in a congestive heart failure clinic: In-hospital time, costs, and patient satisfaction. *Heart & Lung, 12*(3), 237–240.

Clochesy, J., Daley, B., Idemoto, B., Steel, J., Fitzpatrick, J. (1993). Acute care consensus conference (April–May, 1993). Standards for education programs; preparing students as acute care nurse practitioners. *AACN Clinical Issues in Critical Care Nursing, 4,* 593–598.

Crosby, F., Ventura, M.R., Feldman, M.J. (1987). Future research recommendations for establishing NP effectiveness. *Nurse Practitioner, 12*(1), 75–79.

Hooker, R.S., & McCaig, L. (1996). Emergency department uses of physician assistants and nurse practitioners: A national survey. *American Journal of Emergency Medicine, 14,* 245–249.

Keane, A., & Richmond, T. (1993). Tertiary nurse practitioners. *Image Journal of Nursing Scholarship, 25,* 281–284.

Lombness, P. M. (1994). Difference in length of stay with care managed by clinical nurse specialists or physician assistants. *Clinical Nurse Specialist, 8,* 253–260.

McGivern, D. O. The evolution of advanced nursing practice. In Mezy, M. D.

& McGivern, D. O. (Eds.), *Nurses, Nurse Practitioners.* New York: Springer Publishing.

Mitchell-DiCenso, A., Guyatt, G., Marrin, M. et al. (1996). A controlled trial of nurse practitioners in neonatal intensive care. *Pediatrics, 98,* 1143–1148.

Oakland J., & Followell, R.F. (1990). Quality, processes and control. In Statistical Process Control. London: Heineman Newness Publishing.

Piano, M., Kleinpell, R., & Johnson J. (1996). Acute care nurse practitione and management of common health problems. *American Journal of Critical Care, 5*(4), 289–292.

Prescott, P.A., & Driscoll, L. (1979). Nurse practitioner effectiveness. *Evaluation & the Health Professions, 2*(4), 387–418.

Sox, H.C. (1979). Quality of patient care by nurse practitioners and physicians assistants: A ten-year perspective. *Annals of Internal Medicine, 91,* 459–468.

Spisso, J., O'Callaghan, C., McKennan, M., Holcroft, J.W. (1990). Improved quality of care and reduction of house staff workload using trauma nurse practitioners. *The Journal of Trauma, 30*(6), 660–665.

Weinberg, R.M., Lijestrand, J.S., & Moore, S. (1983). Inpatient management by a nurse practitioner: Effectiveness in a rehabilitation setting. *Archives of Physical Medicine Rehabilitation, 64,* 588–590.

Ziemer, D.C., Goldsmith, M.G., Musey, V.C., et al. (1996). Diabetes in urban African Americans. III. Management of type II diabetes in a municipal hospital setting. *American Journal Medicine, 101,* 25–33.

3

Reimbursement, Liability, and Insurance*

Marilyn Hravnak, Margaret Q. Rosenzweig, Deborah Rust, and Kathy Magdic

Acute care nurse practitioners (ACNPs) are more likely to be affiliated with a health care agency or organization than other models of nurse practitioners (NPs) due to the team approach to inpatient care. As such, they are more likely to be employees of an organization or practice plan rather than to provide services to the public as independent agents. It is important that the ACNP and the employer understand the methods for payment for ACNP services under current reimbursement structures and issues related to liability and insurance.

REIMBURSEMENT FOR ACUTE CARE NURSE PRACTITIONER SERVICES

ACNPs and their employers must have an understanding of the market forces shaping their practice. It is imperative that ACNPs be proficient in the specific language related to reimbursement. An overview of cur-

*Thanks are extended to Margaret A. McNeil B.S. Ed. for assistance with manuscript preparation.

rent reimbursement possibilities for all advanced practice nurses precedes those specific to ACNPs. Primarily, reimbursement discussion has focused on Medicare or Medicaid reimbursement from the federal government regulated through the Health Care Finance Association (HCFA) of the Department of Health and Human Services. Traditionally, the large insurance carriers have followed the reimbursement regulations of Medicare or Medicaid. Medicaid is a federally supported, state-administered program that provides health care to certain low income families and dependent children. Medicare covers health-care costs for the elderly or disabled or patients with chronic renal failure. The individual states have wide latitude in the administration of federal money (Mittlestadt, 1993).

Medicaid

Medicaid reimbursement to advanced practice nurse providers varies according to state. Currently all states are under a federal mandate to reimburse pediatric and family NPs providing care to the categorically needy through Medicaid. Reimbursement in this instance is not dependent on physician practice or employing institution. The scope of practice of the NP is defined by the state's nurse practice act. These standard reimbursement rules are changing. If or when Medicaid is administered by block grants to the states, reimbursement mandates for certain populations will no longer be guaranteed. The reimbursement guidelines will need to be redefined on a state by state basis (Sharp, 1996). Increasingly, Medicaid is delivered from within managed care systems or capitated reimbursement structures (May, 1996).

Medicare

Medicare covers costs of hospitals, physicians, and medical services for people more than 65 years of age, disabled persons, and persons with end-stage renal disease. Part A or hospital insurance covers hospital costs. Ninety days of hospital care and 100 days of skilled nursing facility care are allowed. Part A also provides reimbursement to institutions supporting Graduate Medical Education (GME). The GME payments to the hospital are calculated on a per-resident amount reflecting GME costs incurred during a base period and updated by the Consumer Price Index (Federal Register Rules and Regulations, 1995). The moneys are allocated upon base costs of the training program per year. Currently 40 to 50% of the nation's residency programs are funded through Medicare, Part A. Capture of revenue for the services of advanced practice nurses may also occur under Part A when these services are included in the general hospital cost (bed cost) to the patient and are not billed separately (American Nurses Association, 1997). Part B or supplementary medical insurance is paid in monthly premiums by the beneficiary and covers additional medical expenses. Provider costs are included in Part B. Provider services are generally determined based on "visits" or patient encounters per day and billable procedures.

Advanced practice nurses have had increasing reimbursement privileges from Medicare. The first steps were taken in 1990 in an effort at the federal level to increase health-care services to the underserved. These underserved populations included the elderly, rural populations, and patients in federally qualified health centers (Mittlestadt, 1993). At that time, Medicare allowed NPs and clinical nurse specialists (CNSs) to be reimbursed for work in skilled nursing facilities, with reimbursement at 85% of cost made only to the employer of the NP. NPs were not permitted to incorporate and charge for services independently. In 1990, reimbursement for NPs and CNSs serving rural populations in any type of facility in a federally designated rural area was made directly to them or their employer, provided they had a collaborative relationship with a physician (and bound by state interpretation of scope). Reimbursement was the same as for rural health clinics. Medicare benefit was also expanded to the medically underserved in 1990 through the establishment of Federally Qualified Health Centers in order to increase community-based care, as well as prevention, education, and screening services provided by advanced practice nurses (Mittlestadt, 1993). Thus, direct reimbursement to NPs was available only in selected settings and circumstances. At that same time, the services of NPs were also reimbursable as "incident to physician services" in ambulatory care settings if the services followed the plan of care established by the physician and the physician preceptor was on site. Patient encounters and procedures were reimbursed to the physician or practice plan if a contractual relationship was established between the physician and NP at 100% of the physician rate. Direct reimbursement from federally supported programs was not available, however, for NPs in urban, inpatient settings under Part B.

Recently, legislation was passed wherein NPs and CNSs may bill directly for their services under Medicare Part B. The bill was signed into law in August 1997 as H.R. 2105 and went into effect on January 1, 1998. Under this new legislation, NPs may apply for direct reimbursement for services under Medicare Part B regardless of geographic location (Towers, 1997).

The practitioner, working in collaboration with a physician, may be reimbursed at the rate of 80% of the lesser of either the actual charge or 85% of the fee schedule amount of the same services if provided by a physician. NPs serving as assistants at surgery may also be reimbursed at the lesser of the actual charge or 85% of the amount for which a physician serving as assistant to surgery would be eligible (Zimmer, 1997).

Under this new law, a physician does not have to be on site in order for the NP to be eligible for reimbursement. NPs may be reimbursed directly for their services in this situation only if no other facility or provider charges or is paid any amounts for the provision of the services. The same service cannot be billed for simultaneously by the NP and collaborating physician (Sharp, 1997). Likewise, the NPs may not seek support for their services under Part B and still receive redundant full salary support under Part A or facility costs. As in the previous legislation, NPs may also be eligible for reimbursement as "incident to physician services" at 100% of the physician rate (paid only to the physician or employer) when the requirements to be eligible for this type of reimbursement are fulfilled. Each NP must obtain a Medicare Provider Identification Number in order to receive payment. They are permitted to reassign their Medicare benefits to an employer, facility, or health care delivery system if they give permission to do so.

There is a requirement that the NP be working "in collaboration with" a physician in order to be eligible for Medicare reimbursement under the new legislation. This holds true even in states where there is not a requirement for physician collaboration or supervision by statute. As of this date, the clarification of the terms "physician collaboration" and "incident to physician services" had not yet been developed by the Department of Health and Human Services.

Eligibility for direct reimbursement may vary based upon statute. NPs may only apply for services that they are legally authorized to perform within their state's nurse practice act, even though approval may be present at the federal level. Additionally, the interpretation given to the "collaboration" requirement at the federal level may be further abridged if the state has a more restrictive interpretation of, and requirements for, physician collaboration. ACNPs who provide services in the inpatient setting generally already have a collaborative (or even supervisory, depending on the activity) relationship with a physician. The terms of the relationship are outlined in the written practice agreement and the application for clinical privileges. Therefore, the stipulation for such a relationship is likely fulfilled.

It is important to note that, even beyond any revenues they may capture on a fee-for-service basis, ACNPs also significantly enhance the services of the collaborating physician and team and support either added value or cost savings. For example, while the physician is involved in caring for patients with complex, unstable conditions, the ACNP can extend the work of the team by attending to other patients on the service, in the emergency department (ED), on the consult service or in the office. They may also monitor unstable patients closely and implement the plan of care, thereby decreasing the hours the physician may need to be physically present. ACNPs can assess patients prior to rounds, assimilate data, coordinate care, and write notes and orders to lessen the medical workload. The ACNP also provides services to the team that are not afforded by individuals in GME programs. These include their services directed toward care continuity, clinical coordination, enhanced communication, education, and so on. These services result in improved quality, decreased length of stay, and decreased resource use. By acting as the agent to integrate the nursing plan of care with the medical plan of care, a high level of care coordination may be achieved, affecting quality and cost (Parinello, 1995). By facilitating the ability of the attending physician to care for more patients, their potential to increase revenue generation may also be achieved. Cost savings are also facilitated by the thorough documentation practices of ACNPs, which have been noted anecdotally to optimize billing potential.

Because a budgetary analysis may fully indicate their benefit, ACNPs should document the number of individual visits and procedures performed. It is prudent to be able to, on a personal basis, "cost out" their services. The ACNP should keep records indicating workload and know the value of that work in terms of reimbursable dollars as well as through indirect patient care activities. This process will assist ACNPs with future job security, salary negotiation, and improvement of reimbursement strategies (Green & Conway-Welch, 1995)

Private Insurance

Private insurers are varied regarding their policies for advanced practice nursing reimbursement and procedures for obtaining reimbursement. It is important to be familiar with the rules of the company in order to achieve reimbursement to the individual or to the practice. Two large private health plans that currently reimburse advanced practice nurses independently are the Civilian Health and Medical Program of the Uniformed Services (CHAMPUS) and the Federal Employees Health Benefits Program (FEHBP).

Specific Strategies for Obtaining Reimbursement

NPs who wish to use full billing capabilities need to be fluent with computerized billing systems based on a standard diagnostic coding system such as the International Clinical Diagnostic Codes (ICD-9). ICD-9 coding is required for all claims submitted to Medicare (O'Donahue, 1996). It is a World Health Organization classification system. ICD-9 codes are categorized according to diagnosis and severity of illness. There are also mechanisms to code for signs and symptoms, rather than for specific diseases. Therefore, all visits must be coded according to a disease, sign or symptom, and there is no capacity for "rule out" codes. The Physician's Current Procedural Terminology (CPT), established and updated annually by the American Medical Association, must also be used. These are standard descriptions of diagnoses and procedures. Evaluation and Management (E&M) codes are descriptive of visits, including time and complexity. These codes define seven components of inpatient or outpatient visits: history, examination, medical decision making, counseling, coordination of care, nature of the presenting problem, and time. As of this writing, it is felt to be unlikely that new codes will be rewritten in light of the new reimbursement changes for advanced practice nurses. Rather, a modifier to the current coding system will likely be added to designate when the service was performed by an NP or CNS seeking to bill directly for the service.

Diagnostic codes must always accurately reflect the level of service and supplies used to provide the appropriate care. The clinical documentation must scrupulously support the desired codes for appropriate reimbursement and audit (Bryan, 1996). Software is available with coding and HCFA claim forms. Electronic coding is used increasingly, with a significant decrease in overhead costs (Bryan, 1996). ACNPs should, with assistance from the organization, become knowledgeable of codes and terminology in order to accurately reflect the care delivered and secure the most appropriate reimbursement. Their activity in this area has anecdotally optimized accurate revenue capture.

Future Directions in Reimbursement

As noted previously, reimbursement for the services of ACNPs under current reimbursement structures has recently enjoyed increased potential and flexibility. Further reform of health care financing may favor capitated payment systems, however. Under the capitated reimbursement structure, the traditional separation of hospital and provider costs is abandoned. Instead, care is purchased in a "package." The delivery system is integrated to include all services across the health care spectrum: hospital, home care, ambulatory care, and so on. Revenue generated from the enrollees in the plan is divided between these system components. Rather than obtaining fees for individual services, providers are salaried by the payment program. The emphasis is not on volume of patients or numbers of procedures but on cost-effective use of resources to deliver quality care. Under such systems, the financial benefit of ACNPs may be even more directly realized.

Another issue that will affect the future of health care delivery is welfare reform, and it is unknown how this reform will impact advanced practice nursing reimbursement strategies. Most iterations of welfare reconstruction shift the allocation of power away from federal agencies and toward the states. In this situation, the scope of practice as defined by state will most nearly determine the reimbursement potential of NPs. Because fewer individuals will be eligible for welfare, however, the number of those qualified for the associated health benefits will also decrease. This will shrink the reimbursable patient base and leave more individuals without access to health care.

LIABILITY ISSUES

ACNPs should be knowledgeable about their professional liability and insurance protection. Consumers, attorneys, physicians, and health care organizations have become increasingly aware of the use of malpractice claims as a mechanism for the regulation of the quality of health care. The degree to which the NP is held liable for her or his actions is related to the regulations that define accountability and the statute of limitations for nursing malpractice. The regulations that define accountability are discussed in the following chapter. In summary, they include national determination of scope of practice, scope of practice defined by statute (definition for each state), institutional definition of scope (as identified in the institutional scope and standards of practice policy or job description), and scope as identified in the written practice agreement ACNPs develop with collaborating physicians in the inpatient setting. The authority of the NP thus established (and limited by statute) determines the NP's liability (King & Sagan, 1989).

Malpractice

Most law suits for professional malpractice fall within the civil tort category. Tort law is classified as civil injury resulting in breach of legal responsibility from society's expectations (Andrews, Goldberg, & Kaplan, 1996). A professional action resulting in patient harm would characterize this category. If the act of an ACNP is being considered for potential malpractice, three questions may be posed. They are as follows:

What is the nature of the act that is of concern? A court will first determine the nature of the act under question. The act will be judged as to whether it does or does not conform to the expected standards of practice for ACNPs. Liability is established by demonstrating that the care delivery act in question has violated standards of practice or fails to conform to written standards, or both. The assessment of potential violation of nursing standards of practice needs to be established by an advanced nursing practice expert (Eccard & Gainor, 1993). In order to prove neglect or liability in a particular case, the expert witness needs to have educational preparation and clinical background at least equal to the ACNP whose actions are subject to review. Thus it would not be appropriate to have a family NP serve as an expert witness in a case examining the actions of an ACNP.

What are the qualifications of the NP who performed the act? At this point, the court determines if the performance of the act under question requires specific training or knowledge. An ACNP practicing for some time with greater expertise would be expected to conduct his or her actions in a manner appropriate to that level of training and clinical application. For example, if a novice ACNP performs a lumbar puncture without direct supervision and a complication ensues, it would be important to establish how many lumbar punctures this ACNP has performed and the training received pertaining to this procedure (either as a part of the educational program or in postgraduate experiences) (Watts, Hanson, Burke, Gallagher, & Foster, 1996). Failure of the ACNP to exercise appropriate independent judgment in this given situation, in other words, the fact that she or he never had training or previous supervision, would establish her or his liability. If an ACNP who was experienced and expert in the procedure caused a complication, then liability would be examined against compliance with the standard of practice, because educational and clinical preparation would not be in question.

Where was the care provided? The last consideration is related to the setting in which the care is provided. The setting should be able to support the clinical action intended. Within a particular care setting, the types of patient care problems the ACNP is authorized to participate in should be outlined. For example, the practice of an ACNP in a tertiary care setting should be designed so that the ACNP's skills are used effectively but resources are available to support the ACNP and patient care needs if the complexity of the patient's care warrants such assistance (Eccard & Gainor, 1993). The ACNP must be responsible for recognizing his or her practice boundaries (by education, training, or scope of practice) and implementing appropriate communication, referral, or assistance if the situation evolves beyond her or his scope. For instance, if a patient's condition is extremely complex, rapidly changing, or deteriorating, it would be prudent for the ACNP to initiate communication with the collaborating physician. For the ACNP not to do so would be incautious, extending beyond the scope of practice and potentially compromising the patient.

With the three elements outlined, the process of malpractice claim investigation is clear. If the patient was provided the appropriate level of care, the inquiry will focus on the person performing the act. The education and clinical background provide the degree of expertise and skill expected by the ACNP. Establishment of the standard of practice would indicate whether the act in question was nonstandard care. Expert witnesses would evaluate the act in terms adherence to standard care and appropriateness of educational preparation for the action and whether the act was appropriate for the setting.

Professional Liability Coverage

The ACNP has several options available for liability coverage. These include institution or private practice plans and individual plans. The advantages and disadvantages of these coverage options are discussed below.

Employing Institution or Private Practice Plan Insurance

Health care entities (organizations or practice plans) that employ providers carry liability insurance to protect themselves in the event that an error is made by one of their employees. The employer may hold either direct or vicarious liability for the employees' actions. It is recommended that the ACNP obtain a copy of the hospital's or the private practice's insurance policy in order to be aware of their coverage. The ACNP should consider the deductible and threshold limits of the coverage.

Most hospitals carry a maximum dollar coverage that exceeds the basic limit in order to provide them with extra protection. In addition, a deductible provision is carried that makes the hospital responsible for damages under a certain figure. The higher the deductible limit, the lower the premium charged by the insurance company. The ACNP should be aware of the deductible limit because the employer could settle a claim under that amount without consulting the ACNP or the insurer. Such a settlement may reflect negatively upon the ACNP's practice. The ACNP may also face future difficulty in obtaining liability insurance or a new position.

The threshold limit of the coverage should also be considered. Health care institutions are willing to give some control to the insurer to settle cases in their name if the dollar amount sought is below a threshold limit that the insurer and the employer have set, in many instances $3,000. The insurer can choose to settle a claim below the threshold without the employer's permission. Permission from the employer must, however, be obtained in order to settle a case above the threshold. The purpose of the threshold is to protect the employer from having numerous settlements enacted by the insurer without the employer's knowledge, which reflects an unfavorable reputation.

If a claim is placed against the ACNP, the employer's insurance company has the responsibility to provide them with a complete defense, including assigning an attorney to handle the case. Attorney fees, investigation costs and expert witness fees will be paid by the insurer. In the event of a claim, the ACNP should maintain close communication with their employer's legal counsel. ACNPs should be persistent about wanting to be informed throughout the process to insure that decisions made are in their best interest, as well as the interest of the employer.

Individual Professional Liability Insurance

Some NPs believe that purchasing professional liability insurance increases their chances of being sued and makes them a target for compensation claims and that they are adequately covered by the hospital's insurance policy. In personal communication, many attorneys, insurance companies, and NP leaders recommend that the NP carry her or his own professional liability insurance regardless of the setting. It seems, given the discussion of organizational liability coverage previously, that a number of situations might occur in which the ACNP may not wish to be solely dependent on the employer's insurance. Examples might be as follows:

1. The hospital might wish to settle a claim out of court because the dollar amount for compensation would be less than that required for litigation and therefore to the hospital's economic advantage. The ACNP may not be satisfied with having malpractice payments made in her or his name in such a situation, however. The rationale might include preservation of professional integrity or keeping their National Practitioner Data Bank (NPDB) file clean.
2. The employer insurance may settle a claim against the ACNP if the settlement is below the employer's threshold. As previously, the ACNP may have a rationale for not wishing such a settlement against her or his name.
3. The employer may file a claim against the NP if the amount sought in the claim made by the patient is less than the deductible and the employer wishes to recapture those funds. Without liability insurance, even though the NP may successfully challenge such a case and not be held liable for the amount of the claim, the NP may still be liable for court costs accrued in pursuit of this course of action.
4. A claim may be filed against an NP that is not related to misconduct concerning a patient but is related to alleged professional misconduct. For example, a suit may be brought by another provider against the NP for "practicing medicine." Legal costs accrued in addressing such an action would not likely be supported by the employer.
5. NPs may also provide additional services in a setting independent of their hospital practice.
6. The NP may no longer be working at the institution when the claim is made. Retrospective or "tail" coverage may or may not be provided.

A variety of scenarios may thus be possible wherein ACNPs may wish to pursue their own legal counsel and representation. Without professional liability insurance, they are obliged to seek legal opinion autonomously and deal with legal issues in which most ACNPs are not well versed. ACNPs may therefore wish to procure individual professional liability insurance. Such insurance will provide the individual with protection for a specified period of time from the financial consequences of certain professional errors or acts of omission.

When purchasing professional liability insurance, the ACNP should consider both the coverage limits and the type of coverage desired. Policies may provide coverage with "single limits" or "double limits." A single limits policy will provide protection in set dollar increments, for example, $100,000 or $300,000. The stipulated amount will provide protection if a judgment arises out of a single malpractice episode or occurrence that is alleged against the ACNP. In a double limits policy, protection is purchased in a combination package: $100,000/$300,000 or $1,000,000/$3,000,000. The first sum is the amount that is available to the ACNP from a single malpractice occurrence. The larger amount is the maximum amount that will be paid for all policy claims in a given year. The advantage to the double limits policy is that it provides additional dollar coverage in the event of several claims against the ACNP in a single year.

The types of coverage available with individual professional liability insurance come in two forms. These are available in either *occurrence* or *claims-made* policies. The *occurrence policy* covers the ACNP at the time of the act of malpractice. The occurrence policy protects against any incidents that occurred during the time the policy was in effect. Liability protection is provided for events occurring within the period over which the policy was active, even though the claim is filed at a later date (i.e., when the policy may no longer be in effect). A *claims-made policy* provides coverage for claims filed during the effective period of the contract. The claims-made policy is less expensive than an occurrence policy because the risk to the insurance company is less. Even though the action in question occurred during the time the policy was in effect, the insurer is not held accountable if the claim is not made during the active policy period. Statutes of limitation define the time period in which a suit needs to be filed. In some states, the statutes of limitation for medical malpractice claims are shorter than they are for ordinary negligence actions.

Insurance companies offer a wide variety of liability insurance options for NPs. Important steps that ACNPs should take in choosing individual liability insurance that best meets their particular needs include (a) selecting an agent and insurer who is experienced in professional liability insurance, (b) reviewing the extent of the coverage with the agent, (c) inquiring about the types of policies available and understanding the differences, such as claims made versus an occurrence policy, and (d) inquiring about the annual cost of the premium and evaluating the cost of the policy against the protection provided.

The Role of Insurance Companies in a Lawsuit

Professional liability insurance provides the ACNP with financial protection and an attorney or defense counsel. Defense counsel will represent the ACNP during the litigation process. When preparing the defense, the attorney will investigate the subject of the lawsuit, obtain an expert witness, and prepare medical models and the necessary exhibits for the case. There are no costs to the ACNP associated with this process because the cost is incurred by the insurance coverage.

Malpractice litigation can be financially devastating and emotionally agonizing. A lack of knowledge and the limited information in the literature about malpractice liability contributes to the angst. More nurses are being named in lawsuits (Andrews et al., 1996). The courts are beginning to expand the definition of liability as more advanced practice nurses function with increased responsibility and accountability. Becoming more familiar with malpractice law and understanding the implications of professional actions that could lead to a claim are advantageous.

CONCLUSION

ACNPs function in collaboration with physicians, and are generally employees of a healh care delivery entity or practice plan. Both the employee and employer should understand their rights and privileges, as well as their areas of vulnerability when entering the employment relationship. Because the ACNP role is relatively new, it is important that each party have information concerning compensation and liability.

REFERENCES

American Nurses Association. (1997). Medicare and "incident to" payment coverage of nursing services in hospital outpatient clinics and emergency departments. *American Nurses Association Policy Series, No. 96, Pol. 08.* Washington, DC: Author.

Andrews, M., Goldberg, K., & Kaplan, H. (Eds.) (1996). Malpractice liability. *Nurses Legal Handbook* (pp. 201–232). Springhouse, PA: Springhouse Corporation.

Bryan, V. (1996). *Breaking the Code of Health Care Reimbursement with ICD-9–CM.* Leesburg, VA: The Regis Group, Inc.

Eccard, W.T., & Gainor, E.E. (1993). Legal ramifications for expanded practice. In M.D. Mezey & D. O. McGivern (Eds.), *Nurses, Nurse Practitioners: Evolution to Advanced Practice* (pp. 281–321). New York: Springer Publishing Company.

Federal Register Rules and Regulations (1995). Services of residents. *Medicare and Medicaid Guide, Physicians Medicare Fee Schedule, 60*(236), 63141–63148.

Green, A.H., & Conway-Welch, C. (1995). Integrated health care and the advanced practice nurse. *Advanced Practice Nursing Quarterly, 1*(2), 14–21.

King, E. & Sagan, P. (1989). Nurse practitione liability and authority. *Nursing Administration Quarterly, 13*(4): 57–60.

May, C. (1996). States increasingly revamp Medicaid through managed care. *The American Nurse,* October 10.

Mittlestadt, P. (Ed.). (1993). *The Reimbursement Manual; How to Get Paid For Your Advanced Practice Nursing Services* . Washington, DC: American Nurses Association.

O'Donahoe, W. (Ed.). (1996). *Accurate Coding for Critical Care Services and Pulmonary Medicine, 1996* . Northbrook, IL: American College of Chest Physicians.

Parinello, K.M. (1995). Advanced practice nursing: An administrative perspective. *Critical Care Nursing Clinics of North America, 7*(1), 9–16.

Sharp, N. (1997). Fall summary: News from Washington. *The Nurse Practitioner, 22,* 105–112.

Sharp, N. (1996). Nurse practitioner Medicare reimbursement goes to president. *Nursing Management, 1,* 49.

Towers, J. (1997). Medicare reimbursement update. *Academy Update; American Academy of Nurse Practitioners,* 13(7):1.

Watts, R.J., Hanson, J.S., Burke, K.G., Gallagher, S.M., & Foster, D.E. (1996). The critical care nurse practitioner: An advanced practice role for the critical care nurse. *Dimensions of Critical Care Nursing, 15,* 48–56.

Zimmer, P.A. (1997). Opening the gate: Direct Medicare reimbursement for NPs. *NP Directions, 2*(1):3.

4

Scope of Practice, Credentialing, and Privileging

Marilyn Hravnak, Margaret Q. Rosenzweig, Deborah Rust, and Kathy Magdic

Nurse practitioners (NPs) are finding increased job opportunities in the acute care setting. As a greater need is recognized, educational programs specifically designed to prepare acute care nurse practitioners (ACNPs) have evolved, and an ACNP national certification exam is now available. As compared with other models of NPs (family, adult, and pediatric NPs), the ACNP is more likely to be affiliated with a health care agency, organization, or physician practice plan rather than engaged in an independent practice. This is due to the complex health problems patients within this specialty experience and the collaborative team approach to inpatient care. It is imperative that the ACNP and the employer consider a variety of factors to optimize the organizational framework within which the ACNP will be employed. This chapter will discuss organizational considerations related to ACNP practice, including (1) preparation of the health care organization to recognize and use ACNP talents maximally and (2) preparation of the ACNP to function as an agent of the employer in the provision of patient care. Addressing the organizational and individual issues proactively will help to ensure successful establishment and growth of this newest advanced practice nursing role.

ORGANIZATIONAL PREPARATION FOR ACUTE CARE NURSE PRACTITIONER PRACTICE

Development of the Vision and the Model

The organization should first examine the motivation for implementing the ACNP role and the institutional needs the ACNPs are expected to fill. Downsizing of house staff is cited as one of the rationales for needing ACNPs (Dracup et al., 1994; Richmond & Keane, 1996; Spisso, O'Callaghan, McKennan, & Holcroft, 1990). Although diminished numbers of medical trainees within the inpatient setting contribute an impetus, the rationale for hiring ACNPs should not be to have the same functions performed in the same manner as with house staff. Recently, Ford (1997), founder of the NP movement, was asked to reflect on the genesis and evolution of the role. She noted that a deficit of physicians available to provide pediatric services in rural Colorado in 1965 contributed to the need that she expected NPs to fill. The goal was not to replace physicians but to implement an advanced role for nurses, and the physician deficit provided the opportunity to test the new role's efficacy. Likewise, ACNPs should not be marketed or used solely as "resident replacements." Such an approach might fill the medical trainee gap but would not use the unique skills and talents that are part of the NP role and also congruent with the types of outcomes that organizations are currently seeking.

The model should instead incorporate role responsibilities that contribute to current patient and organizational needs that ACNPs have been educated to accomplish. Certainly the ACNP functions as a direct provider of quality care, diagnosing and managing health care problems of the acutely and critically ill within a collaborative framework. The ACNP also provides for continuity of care because, unlike residents or interns, they do not rotate through clinical services. In addition, they perform services for which nurses are especially skilled, such as communication with patients and families; educating patients, families and staff; facilitating the movement of patients through the system; and patient advocacy. ACNPs are also prepared to facilitate managed care modalities, develop and implement protocols and critical pathways and apply cost-effective strategies and resource conservation. Some of the role responsibilities of ACNPs are related to the health promotion and protection basis to their practice, a foundation that is shared with other NP specialties (Hravnak & Magdic, 1997). In the acute care setting, the ACNPs' health promotion activities strongly focus on risk factor identification and minimization. They are qualified to identify problems for which the inpatient population is at risk and to implement strategies to minimize or prevent risk. Many of the health risks for which the ACNP monitors inpatients and intervenes are physiological in nature. These physiological risks include immobility, diminished nutrition, fluid and electrolyte imbalance, altered immunocompetence, existing or developing comorbid conditions, and risks imposed by the invasive nature of our diagnostic and treatment modalities. Other risks have a more psychological basis; still others result from a multiplicity of caregivers and fragmentation of services (Hravnak and Magdic, 1997). This health promotion and protection focus of the ACNP's practice fills patient and organizational needs for prevention of complications and increased patient (and staff) well being, making the ACNP a unique and desirable commodity in the marketplace. In summary, the ACNP provides services that have not been provided by residents, such as continuity of patient care, clinical coordination (Parinello, 1995), and health promotion and protection. Their addition to the provider team is thus a service enhancement rather than a service replacement and represents value added.

When the health-care entity evaluates organizational needs, it is equally important to question whether or not the ACNP role is best suited to meet the needs. The bulk of job responsibilities for ACNPs is with direct patient care provision, health promotion and protection, and clinical coordination. If the organizational needs are more heavily related to teaching, supporting, and educating the nursing staff; conducting research; developing organization-wide policies and systems; or supervising staff, then a clinical nurse specialist, nurse researcher or nurse administrator might be a better choice. Although aspects of these activities are components of the ACNPs education and role, they are not the major focus. Not choosing the right "fit" will result in dissatisfaction for the employer and ACNP, as well as role diffusion.

Identifying and Putting Into Operation the Scope of Practice

Once the need has been identified and the ACNP role determined to best meet the need, then the scope of practice for the ACNP within the organization or agency can be more concretely described (Hravnak, Rosenzweig, & Baldisseri, 1996). The scope of practice for each ACNP is derived from five sources, which are illustrated in Figure 4.1.

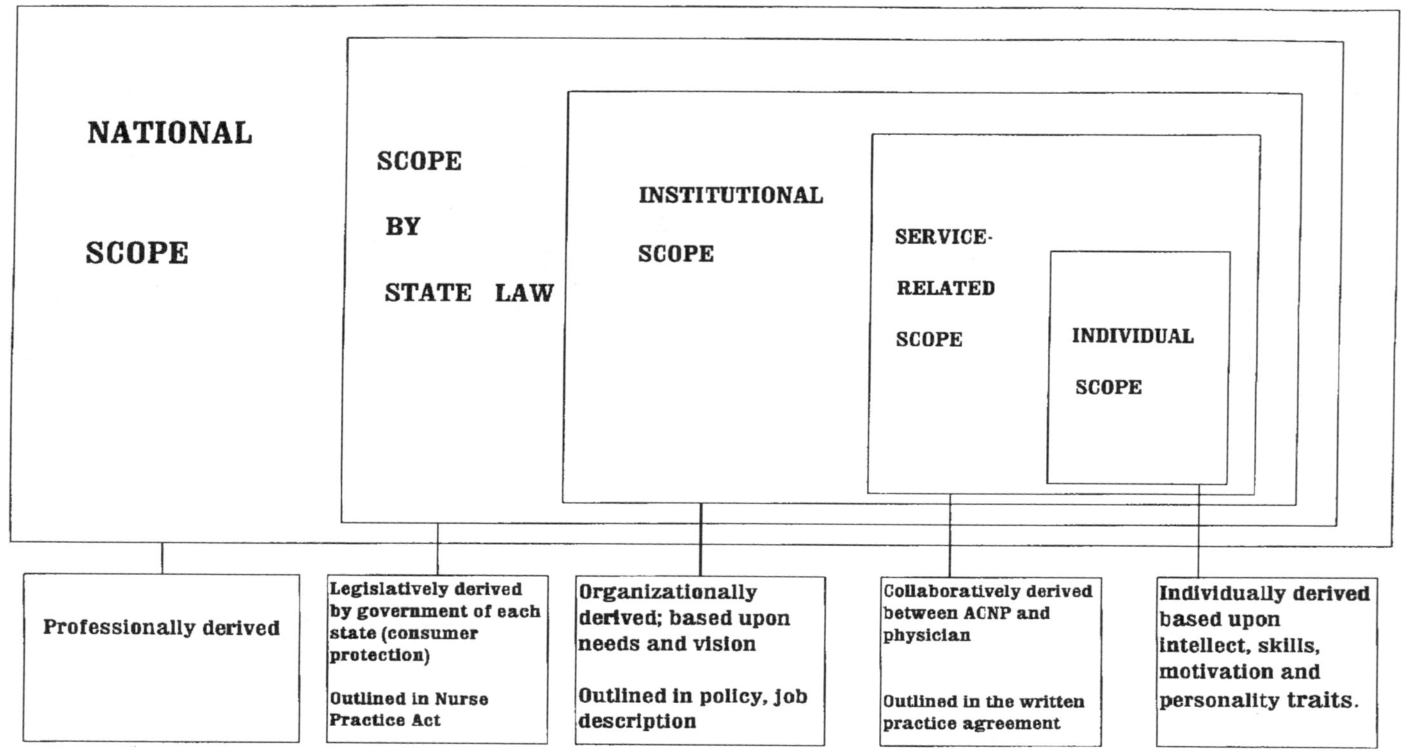

FIGURE 4.1 Derivation of each individual acute care nurse practitioner's (ACNP's) scope of practice.

National Standards

The *Standards of Clinical Practice and Scope of Practice for the Acute Care Nurse Practitioner* (American Nurses Association, 1995) was developed collaboratively by the American Nurses Association and the American Association of Critical Care Nurses. This document delineates the scope of ACNP practice in broad terms. The breadth is necessary to provide for future growth of the role and variations in scope that result from individual modifications in each state's nurse practice act. In defining the scope of the ACNP's practice, the document identifies the ACNP's purpose as the provision of advanced nursing care across the continuum of acute care services to patients who are acutely and critically ill using a collaborative model. Care provision should be comprehensive and uninterrupted and may be provided in a variety of settings (i.e., not limited to the traditional hospital setting). The document identifies restorative care as the focus of the ACNP practice. The ACNP's short-term goal is patient stabilization, provision of physical and psychological care, and minimization of complications, whereas the long-term goal is restoration of the patient's maximal health potential (with concurrent evaluation of risk factors in achieving this outcome). The Standards of Care outlined in this document are organized according to the nursing process and provide the framework for the ACNP's practice with respect to assessment, diagnosis, outcome identification, planning, implementation, and evaluation. The Standards of Professional Performance describe the ACNPs role in the areas of quality of care, performance appraisal, education, collegiality, ethics, collaboration, research, and resource use. The constraints of this chapter do not permit a comprehensive interpretation of the national ACNP scope of practice. Organizations who have or will be employing the services of ACNPs are encouraged to use the document, however.

Statutes

The government, representing individual citizen consumers of health care services, also influences a professional's scope of practice. The government defines nurses' scope of practice and prevents inappropriate individuals from practicing through licensure statutes. In the nurse practice act, the state delineates educational requirements and the types of activities that may be performed by those granted permission to use the title (Hall, 1993). Currently, advanced practice nurses are not licensed beyond their registered nurse license. In most states, however, one must provide evidence of additional qualifications to practice in the expanded role of a NP with title protection. This activity is covered under a registration or certification statute and is not a licensure statute (Hall, 1993). Both licensure and registration or certification statutes differ from state to state, as well as differing from agency to agency within the federal government (Gilliam, 1994). In some states advanced practice nursing is administered solely by the Board of Nursing, whereas in others there is joint administration by the Boards of Nursing and Medicine. Some states do not have a requirement for supervision of the NP by a physician; others do. There are also varying degrees of prescriptive authority granted to NPs by statute (Pearson, 1995, 1996, 1997). Health care organizations will want to contact their Board of Nursing to access the scope for NPs in their state and determine the qualifications necessary to perform the role. It is helpful to secure an annotated copy of the nurse practice act, wherein each section includes notations describing cases that interpret each section. It is usually possible to obtain an annotated version of the state's nurse practice act from a state senator or representative or a law library (Hall, 1993). In states where NP practice is jointly promulgated by the nursing and medicine boards, it is helpful to obtain a copy of the Medical Practice Act. Practice acts are broad in scope. Most states do not differentiate between NP practice specialties (family practice, adult, pediatric, acute care, etc.). They will not provide a "laundry list" of skills, tasks, or procedures permissible within the scope. In trying to examine the practice act to determine what an ACNP "can and cannot" do within their scope, it is best to interpret the act as broadly as possible (assume "can" unless "cannot" is described) and give plain and ordinary meaning to the words used in the statute. It is frequently helpful to request the assistance of the hospital's legal counsel with the interpretation. Some ACNPs may be disheartened by the restrictive nature of their practice acts. Organizations and health care agencies will not be willing to support the practice of NPs beyond their state-defined scope, however, due to the legal responsibility they bear as employers.

Institutional Standards

Although professional and state determinations of scope will provide a base, the institutional definition will more clearly delineate the patient population the ACNP is hired to serve, the needs to be filled, the knowledge base required, and the process for collaboration with the other health care providers in the institution (Parinello, 1995). Institutional determination of scope may be set forth in a job description, a hospital policy, or both.

Service-Related Standards

The ACNP's scope of practice may be further delineated based on the needs of a specific patient population or care delivery team within the organization. The service related scope of practice is derived by the individual ACNP, collaborating physician, and nurse administrator. The terms of service-related scope are set forth in the written practice agreement. For example, an NP with an orthopedic surgery service may have responsibility for cast removal; an ACNP in an intensive care unit may place central lines; the NP on the renal medicine service may write orders for hemodialysis; the NP with cardiology may initiate treatment regimens for patients experiencing dysrhythmias other than those covered under Advanced Cardiac Life Support recommendations; the NP with the cardiothoracic surgery team may have first-assist responsibilities in the operating room. Actions specific to the service-related scope of practice should be detailed in the written practice agreement.

Individual Standards

Scope of practice is lastly determined by the knowledge base and talents of the individual ACNP. Prior experience, specialization, motivation, self-esteem, personal ethics, personality traits, and communication style contribute to the ACNP's intellectual and technical skill set. The individual must seek ongoing education. The ACNP must be knowledgeable of recent advances published in the medical and nursing literature and evaluate research for potential application to practice. The ACNP must truly accept the invitation to become a life-long learner, because quality and safety of patient care depend on it.

The process of deriving the scope of practice and standards for the ACNP within the organization is summarized as follows: First, determine the scope of practice using the professionally generated national scope of ACNP practice as the basis and perform a cross-check against advanced practice nursing registration or certification statutes for further circumscription. The scope should then be refined (based on identified organizational needs) to characterize the institutional ACNP scope of practice within a job description or policy. Institutional performance standards for ACNP practice are then developed from the institutional scope of practice. The national standards of practice should be used as the basis and modified to reflect the operation of the institutional scope of practice. The practice standards thus derived and included in the job description provide the platform for performance evaluation and outcome measurement (Parinello, 1995). Lastly, the ACNP, physician, and nurse administrator should outline the ACNP's intended actions that are unique to a particular patient population or service team in the written practice agreement.

Job Description and Written Agreement

The job description is the operation of the health care agency's scope and standards for ACNP practice. The job description should summarize the scope of practice, list job qualifications, and outline the communication and "reporting" mechanism. The performance standards within the job description describe the responsibilities for which the ACNP is accountable and provide a template against which both the practitioner and the employer can evaluate performance. They should be written using measurable criteria and reflect outcomes for the patient, the organization, and the professional practice. One comprehensive job description should be written to encompass the practice of all ACNPs within the organization, regardless of the area or department in which they work or the specialty patient population served. Having one job description promotes consistency and congruence in the understanding and application of the role across the organization by the myriad personnel with whom the ACNP interacts. The job description should typify the end product, describing performance standards and the degree of responsibility and accountability that one would expect a seasoned, expert ACNP to maintain. Details related to specific tasks and the specialty patient population are best accommodated in the written practice agreement.

A written practice agreement describes the clinical functions and tasks of the individual ACNP and the medical regimens that may be administered or relayed by her or him (Burkholder & Dudjak, 1994). Both the ACNP and collaborating physician specifically describe and agree to the type of activities the ACNP will perform as a member of the practice or team. They also prescribe the level of communication between the ACNP and the physician prior to performance of specific functions. One purpose of the written agreement is for the ACNP and collaborating physician to achieve a level of detail and specificity in describing clinical functions not attained in the job description. It also ensures that both the ACNP and the physician consent to the inclusion of these tasks within the ACNP's scope of practice and communicates the agreement to other team members. Also, the physician may carry some vicarious liability for the ACNP's practice as either her or his employer or where statute requires that the NP practice with physician direction or supervision. In these cases, the written practice agreement ensures that both parties clearly understand the extent of the ACNP's duties. Additionally, the written practice agreement provides a mechanism for the upward titration of the responsibilities of the ACNP as she or he progresses from novice to expert. As the ACNP becomes increasingly skilled over time, the level of autonomy in performing clinical functions progresses. As new skills become available (i.e., through technological advancement) or necessary (i.e., a different patient population will be served by the team) they may be added to the list. Lastly, the written agreement serves as the basis for the application for clinical privileges. Further discussion follows.

PREPARING THE INDIVIDUAL FOR THE ORGANIZATION

After the ACNP is employed, a variety of steps need to be undertaken to smoothly assimilate the ACNP into organizational operations. The ACNP should be oriented to the organizational philosophy, mission, and structure. The ACNP should also be oriented to the patient care delivery system and departmental responsibilities. The ACNP must understand the operation of the organization's systems in order to support role aspects related to clinical coordination and indirect care provision.

A variety of organizational models may be used for ACNP implementation. In one model, the ACNP is positioned solely within the nursing department and structure. In this model, the ACNP reports to nursing administrators. Although the nursing administrators collaborate with physicians regarding the clinical functions of the ACNP, organizational functions such as system coordination and indirect care services are determined entirely by nursing. Another choice is to position the ACNP role within the physician practice plan. This model strengthens the clinical focus of the ACNP and has the advantage of frequent and ongoing communication and goal establishment between the ACNP and the physician partners. A disadvantage may be lack of understanding or support of the professional nursing focus and organizational aspects and a tendency for the communication to become hierarchical (physician down to nurse employee) rather than relational (between partners). Another model is a blended or hybrid model (Parinello, 1995) that emphasizes joint practice. In this model, the nurse and physician are equal partners. The physician's decision takes precedence when the issue is more closely related to medicine, and the ACNP's decision takes precedence when the issue is more closely related to nursing. In the hybrid model, the ACNP generally has two reporting mechanisms—through medicine and nursing. An advantage to this model is the full use of the nursing and medical strength brought to the partnership. A disadvantage, common to other matrix reporting relationships, is the potentially variant expectations of physician and nursing supervisors, resulting in a lack of clear identification of priorities or function. Regardless of the model chosen, it is imperative that the ACNP be clear about lines of communication, procedures for conflict resolution, mechanisms for measurement of outcome variables, and the procedures and individuals involved in performance evaluations.

Credentialing and Privileging

The ACNP must participate in credentialing and privileging processes in order to provide care as an agent of the hospital. Although conducted simultaneously, credentialing and privileging are two separate operations with different meanings and intent. *Credentialing* delineates a process whereby the professional and technical competence of a licensed provider is formally recognized by an agency, institution, or organization (Kristeller, 1995). *Privileging* is the process whereby the medical staff or credentialing committee evaluates and recommends that an individual practitioner be permitted to provide specific clinical functions within the hospital (Dent, 1996). An individual may be capable by preparation, license, and practice history to perform certain acts (credentialed), but they may not be granted permission by the hospital to provide these services to the hospital's clients (privileged).

The hospital is provided with significant impetus to establish initial and ongoing competence of providers within the organization and control the types of services that they provide. This impetus is provided by both the legal and the ethical liability the hospital assumes for delivery of quality care to its clients and requirements by regulatory agencies.

Establishing the Rationale for Credentialing and Privileging

ACNPs should be aware of the circumstances that provide the rationale for credentialing and privileging and that compel the organization to develop systems for their accomplishment. This background includes liability law and requirements imposed on the organization by regulatory agencies.

Liability Law. It has been clearly established that hospitals and their component medical staffs may be held liable for damages if they permit an unqualified physician to practice within the confines of the hospital (Harty-Golder, 1993). This principle has been upheld in numerous court decisions, such as Darling v. Charleston Memorial Hospital (1965, 1966); Purcell v. Zimbelman (1972); and Mitchell v. Joiner (1971). More recently, the courts have extended this responsibility to include liability in the event the credentials of physicians newly admitted to the staff are not adequately investigated or for failure to sufficiently monitor the quality of treatment delivered by a physician while practicing at the hospital, as in Arthur v. St. Peter's Memorial Hospital (Laws Div. 1975) (Benesch, 1993). Failure of the hospital to use reasonable care to verify education, training, and experience prior to appointment to the medical staff is considered a breach of duty to the public (Benesch, 1994). If the breach of duty results in injury to a patient, the hospital will be liable for damages incurred (Johnson v. Misericordia Community Hospital [1981]; Ferguson v. Gonyaw [1976]). A hospital is also bound to remove a staff member where there is notice of incompetence, as in Corleto v. Shore Memorial Hospital (1975). There are three conditions under which the hospital may be held liable for the actions of providers. The first is respondeat superior, which holds employers secondarily (vicariously) responsible for the actions of their employees where the employer has the right to control the work and the employee is acting within his or her scope of practice. The second possible condition of vicarious liability is that of ostensible agency. This situation is very similar to respondeat superior. In this situation, however, the provider has been viewed as an employee of the agency, even though he or she is not. The third situation is that of corporate liability, wherein the organization has its own professional duty directly owed to its clients. The duties of selecting medical staff and supervising or monitoring their actions are two duties of the health care agency held to be nondelegable (Benesch, 1994). Although the medical staff participates in the process as indicated in the hospital bylaws, the organization holds the ultimate authority and liability.

Because hospitals are increasingly held liable for services provided by physicians on the hospital premises, hospitals are now given more latitude to ensure that the credentials of those seeking privileges are adequate and that the quality of care delivered within the facility is safe. The law thus provides an inducement for hospitals to use reasonable care to develop systems to verify the credentials of physicians seeking to practice in the institution, recredential them yearly, and revoke the privilege to practice when a breach of duty or serious question concerning care delivery is raised (Benesch, 1993). In addition to physician and dentist providers, others who deliver medical care and must be credentialed and apply for clinical privileges within the hospital include independently licensed providers such as podiatrists and psychologists and "dependent practitioners" such as NPs and physician assistants.

Regulatory Agencies. The information above provides the legislative rationale supporting credentialing and privileging activities; further requirements are imposed upon the hospital to develop systems for credentialing and privileging by regulatory agencies. These regulatory agencies include the National Practitioner Data Bank (NPDB), operated by the Health, Resources and Services Administration (HRSA), and the Joint Commission for the Accreditation of Health Care Organizations (JCAHO).

The NPDB was formed as a result of federal legislation. The Health Care Quality Improvement Act (P.L. 99-660) was passed in 1986, followed by the Medicare and Medicaid Patient and Program Protection Act in 1987 (Birkholz, 1991; Culbertson, 1991). Under the Health Care Quality Improvement Act, the HRSA was mandated to develop a national registry of providers (physicians, dentists, and other health care practitioners) who lose malpractice claims and those who are subject to adverse actions of greater than 30 days on licensure, privileges, or society memberships (Ankney, Coil, Kolff, & Esper, 1995). The federal repository for this information is the NPDB, which began operation on September 1, 1990 (Birkholz, 1991). The intent of the data bank is to provide potential employers with timely information about adverse actions against health care providers, thereby limiting the ability of such individuals to endanger the public by transferring from state to state without disclosing such information (Birkholz, 1991; Gabel, 1993).

Conditions that must be reported to the NPDB are noted in Table 4.1. Significant monetary sanctions are imposed on hospitals, insurers, professional boards, and professional societies who do not comply with the reporting requirements. For instance, a civil penalty of up to $10,000 for each failure to report malpractice payment may be imposed. Additionally, a hospital that does not report actions against the license or clinical privileges of an individual loses its immunity to liability for the deeds of that professional. The hospital is also liable for the malpractice of a provider if they fail to query the data bank and discover information that would have resulted in denial of clinical privileges on hire (i.e., they did not exert reasonable care in assuring competency).

Hospitals are required to query the NPDB when a provider makes an application for medical staff appointment or clinical privileges and every 2 years thereafter. Other entities who may query the data bank include state licensing boards, other health care entities, professional societies, the plaintiff's attorney, and a health care practitioner (own file only) (Birkholz, 1995).

A second agency that supports formation of organizational credentialing and privileging processes is the JCAHO. Since January 1, 1989, the JCAHO has established standards requiring the extensive report of risk management, quality assurance, peer review, and credentialing functions. They define credentialing as the process of granting authorization by the governing body to provide specific patient care and treatment services in the hospital, within defined limits, based on an individual's license, education, training, experience, competence, heath status, and judgment (Hershey, 1994). In order to meet these standards, hospitals must develop mechanisms to gather information concerning these activities and provide links to collate, compile, and evaluate the information obtained. The standards require that information gained on the medical staff application be verified with the primary sources. Second, medical staff bylaws rules and regulation must stipulate the circumstances in which a practitioner must report actions taken against professional liability. The JCAHO further requires that a mechanism be in place to collect specific information (previous or current) related to actions affecting licensure, registration, adjustment, or termination or clinical privileges. Last, the information just outlined is required to be updated and reviewed prior to reappointment.

Contingencies may result if compliance to the above standards is lacking (Shala, 1991). The JCAHO also has guidelines for the granting and renewal of privileges to practice on the hospital's medical staff. Privi-

TABLE 4.1 Actions That Must Be Reported to the National Practitioner Data Bank

Action	Comment
Malpractice Settlements	Any malpractice settlement must be reported by the person or entity making payment, regardless of the dollar amount (Birkholz, 1991). Only requirements are that payment is made on the behalf of the professional and a written claim or complaint requesting payment exists.
	Proof of wrongdoing is not necessary. Does not make a difference if the payment is made as a result of action determined by trial (in court) or in settlement made before trial (out of court) (Gabel, 1993). Even cases settled by the insurance carrier because there was an economic advantage to presettle when compared with the cost of litigation (so-called "nuisance cases") are also reportable.
	Within 30 days of payment, a report must be made to the NPDB and the professional board in the state where the alleged event occurred.
	Reports on malpractice payments made on behalf of advanced practice nurses are required by this legislation.
Clinical Privileges	Only adverse actions that influence clinical privileges for greater than 30 days duration are reportable. These actions include denial, decrease, or revocation of clinical privileges when prompted by incompetence.
	Voluntary surrender of privileges when such surrender occurs in response to threat of investigation or in exchange for withholding investigation is also reportable. Surrender of privileges in response to situations not related to an individual patient's welfare (i.e., change of job description or location, change in services provided by the hospital) is not reportable. Censure and reprimands are not reportable (Birkholz, 1991).
	Actions against the clinical privileges of NPs are not required to be reported to the NPDB currently, but hospitals may do so.
	In the event action is taken on an NP's clinical privileges, notice is sent to the state board of medical examiners within 15 days of final action, which in turn reports to the NPDB and the state nursing board within 15 days of receipt.
Licensure Actions	Adverse action against a nurses license that is a result of formal review is reportable. Censure, reprimands, denials, revocations, and restrictions to licenses are all reportable (Birkholz, 1991).

TABLE 4.1 *Continued*

	Licensure actions are reportable only after final action has been taken.
	If the professional has voluntarily entered a substance abuse program and was not asked to surrender his or her license, the event is not reportable under this section (but if clinical privileges are curtailed, it may be reportable under the previous section). If the rehabilitation program is not successfully completed and the board takes formal action, then the revocation is reported.
Professional Society Memberships	Actions that result in revocation of professional society membership are optionally reportable.

leges are based on training and experience, health status, and quality of care (Benesch, 1994). JCAHO has further determined that it is the hospital's responsibility to ensure that nonphysician providers are qualified and competent to provide patient care. They charge the governing body of the hospital with this responsibility, but permit delegation of the management of the systems required to achieve this goal to the medical staff or administrative departments (Gilliam, 1994).

Note that there is congruence between the information that the JCAHO requires and the information that must be forwarded to the NPDB. Thus, the JCAHO prescribes that each hospital develop a system to scrutinize the qualifications and competence of those seeking to practice upon hire and systematically thereafter (credentialing and privileging). Misconduct recognized through implementation of this system is then forwarded to the NPDB (Hravnak & Baldisseri, 1997).

The Process of Credentialing and Privileging Acute Care Nurse Practitioners

Frequently, ACNPs are credentialed and privileged by the organization using the same system that is in place for physicians. When a larger number of ACNPs hired by the hospital warrants it, however, a separate system or structure to support their credentialing and privileging may be implemented if the hospital board delegates this authority to such an entity. Since credentialing and privileging is a form of peer review, advanced practice nurses must have representation on committees that review the qualifications and privilege requests of other advanced practice nurses; otherwise the "peer" criterion is not fulfilled and nursing qualifications are reviewed by nonnurses.

As noted earlier, *credentialing* provides the hospital with a system whereby the professional and technical competence of the ACNP may be ascertained. The credentials that the ACNP will need to provide are listed in Table 4.2. In summary, they include proof of initial and ongoing education, licensure, and certification. In the effort to document ongoing technical competence, the ACNP should keep and submit a record of skill performance (type, number, complication rate). Because the professional references will be asked to attest to the *observed* clinical competence and ethical integrity of the individual seeking credentialing, it is best to choose an individual who has worked closely with the ACNP in a clinical capacity. The falsification of any information on the application, including the request for report of action against licensure or priv-

TABLE 4.2 Credentials That ACNPs Provide to Health Care Organizations for Credentialing and Requests for Clinical Privileges

Proof of education (a transcript may be requested)
Copy of RN license
Copy of state-issued documentation granting the title to practice as an advanced practice nurse (in states where provided)
DEA number (if applicable)
Certification (not universally required, always preferred)
Clinical practice experience
Clinical references
Actions against license
Action against privileges
Disciplinary action
Professional activities
Continuing education
Current life support certification
If "on call" requests are part of the job, demonstration of ability to respond within a certain time frame
Proof of malpractice insurance may be requested
A sponsoring physician(s)
A written agreement between the ACNP and the sponsoring physician
Practice protocols
A list of the practice privileges being requested, including supervision parameters as necessary

Note. From "Credentialing and privileging: Insight into the process," by Hravnak, M., & Baldisseri M., 1997, *AACN Clinical Issues, 8,* 113. Reprinted with permission.

ileges and previous disciplinary action, is grounds for immediate dismissal.

JCAHO requires that the credentials be verified with the primary source and that the date and result of the verification be documented. The American Medical Association keeps an extensive data base of practicing physicians, including progress through medical school and postgraduate training programs, states where they are licensed to practice, actions taken by state licensing boards, and information from the Drug Enforcement Agency. The JCAHO now permits hospitals to use this information in place of primary source verification for physicians (Brandt, 1996). Since no such data base exists for advanced practice nurses, primary source verification must take place. The record of verification must be kept with the application and include name of inquirer, date of inquiry, contact person, and substance of the response (Harty-Golder, 1993). The credentialing process may take weeks to months. Reappointment to the staff may be made on a periodic basis (generally biannually), and pertinent portions of the credentialing process (verification of continuing education) may require reverification.

Within the *privileging* process, the medical staff or credentialing committee evaluates an individual practitioner and recommends that he or she be permitted to provide specific patient care services within the hospital (Hravnak & Baldisseri, 1997; Smith, 1993; Smith, 1991). By "delineating clinical privileges," the hospital will determine which diagnostic or therapeutic procedures the practitioner may perform (or order) and which conditions they may treat within well-defined limits (Kristeller, 1995). The types of privileges conferred, and their limits, are in part based on the individual practitioner's professional license and scope of practice, documented training, experience, competence, health status, and patient population. In the case of the ACNP, they may also be related to the practice and patient population served by the collaborating physician. Privileges conferred may also be related to the mission and goals of the hospital. Even though an individual is educationally qualified and licensed (and even have documented clinical proficiency in the skill) he or she may not necessarily be granted the privilege to perform the skill by the hospital or be permitted to render this type of care to the hospital's clientele. The goals of the privileging process include (but are not limited to) the assurance of high-quality patient care, minimization of the hospital's legal risk, and fulfillment of the hospital's mission (Hravnak & Baldisseri, 1997).

Because ACNPs generally develop a written practice agreement with a collaborating physician, the list of privileges requested may be culled from the agreement. They are generally limited to clinical functions, tasks, and procedures. Procedures may be compartmentalized into minor procedures and invasive procedures. The privilege to act as first or second assistant in the operating room should be requested if pertinent. Privileges to order specific therapies such as hyperalimentation or blood product administration may be delineated, as well as hemodialysis or renal replacement therapy. Some institutions may request that the degree of physician consultation (or supervision) be specified for certain conditions or actions. The services that the credentialed practitioner is privileged to provide may change over time. Further training, evolution of clinical mastery, and increase in the types of services provided by the hospital or team may warrant expansion of privileges. The individual's privilege to practice in a closely supervised manner may expand to a more autonomous level of performance as safe repetition of the acts or skills are demonstrated. Alternatively, an individual may experience withdrawal of privileges to perform certain acts or skills if the hospital eliminates or curtails the service, ongoing competency cannot be demonstrated (perhaps due to inadequate exposure or opportunity for repetition), or as a response to internal disciplinary action. (Only the last situation requires report to the NPDB). Generally, re-examination and reissue of the clinical privileges granted occurs on an annual or biannual basis.

A debate currently exists in the literature with respect to proving ongoing technical competency. Individuals are questioning the number of procedures that must be performed in a given time period to constitute or verify competency (Eliason, 1994; Grumet, 1993; Mussalam, 1995; Susman & Rodney, 1994). It is not clear that "numbers equal competency," and some believe that competency should be measured by demonstrated ability rather than by quotas that may not have scientific validity (Norris & Susman, 1995).

A summary of the events in the process for credentialing and privileging a provider to provide services within the health care organization are listed in Table 4.3. Outside the hospital setting, credentialing and privileging requirements may also exist for providers contracting with HMOs. The fact that a physician or NP is listed by the HMO as an approved provider infers to subscribers that his or her credentials are acceptable to the HMO. Public policy encourages that HMOs be found vicariously

TABLE 4.3 Events Constituting the Process of Credentialing and Privileging

The ACNP files an application
The information within the application (see Table 4.2) is verified with the primary source
Inquiry to the NPDB is made
Information regarding past or impending lawsuits, withdrawal or curtailment of clinical privileges, or disciplinary action is investigated
Delineation of clinical privileges is determined (based on written practice agreement)
Recommendations are forwarded by the entity conducting credentialing and privileging (medical staff, credentialing committee, etc.) to the hospital board
Final approval is granted
Credentials and requested privileges are reviewed and recommended on an ongoing basis (usually annually or biannually)

liable for negligence by their individual providers. HMOs might not have sufficient incentive to select and retain providers with the best credentials without such an expectation (Benesch, 1994). HMOs are therefore increasingly credentialing and privileging providers within their plans. ACNPs in collaborative relationships with physician practice plans that contract with HMOs may therefore still be subject to a credentialing and privileging process (wherein approval rests with the HMO), even though they may not see inpatients.

Economic Credentialing

A current trend is the concept of economic credentialing (Price, 1993). This trend is to some degree stimulated by the current managed care environment, wherein financial risk is shared by the payer (the health maintenance organization or HMO) and the provider (hospital and clinician). In order to develop and retain a contract with the payer, hospitals are challenged to provide high-quality care. They must do so while maintaining cost efficiency, productivity, and provident resource use, however, in order to maintain solvency. The payer organization examines the provider organization as a whole to assess these outcomes (Stahl, 1995). Increasingly, provider organizations are noting each individual practitioner's singular contribution to its aggregate outcomes. The use of economic criteria as additional factors in making clinical appointment and privileging decisions is a reflection of the business orientation evolving in health care (Hershey, 1994). Individual health-care entities (independent of their affiliations with payer organizations) are getting some support for adding economic criteria to their evaluation of individuals for appointment, reappointment, and privileging. One court case involved a cardiac surgeon (Rosenblum) and a medical center (Tallahassee Memorial Regional Medical Center). The physician in question was head of an open heart surgery program at one hospital, and had requested appointment and clinical privileges at a second competing hospital. In that case, the second appointment was denied on economic grounds. There was a fear on the part of the second hospital that all the surgeon's high risk patients might be forwarded to them, and the court concluded that the hospital board had a fiduciary responsibility to protect the interests and assets of the hospital (Hudson, 1993).

Within economic credentialing, individuals applying or reapplying for credentialing and granting of clinical privileges are assessed using a dimension of economic efficiency, in addition to the traditional indicators of professional and technical competence (Benesch, 1993). Some of the specific measures of economic efficiency by which a clinician might be evaluated could include length of stay by diagnosis related group (DRG), charges per admission by DRG, charges or length of stay adjusted for severity of illness, utilization review denials by third party payers, bad debt or write offs, malpractice settlements, timely medical record completion, and incident reports (Kolb, Hughes, & Young, 1993). Somc hospitals use profiling systems that facilitate assessment of an individual's performance over a given time period. These profiles include clinical as well as economic performance measures, and the profiles can be evaluated for credentialing purposes (Blum, 1995).

Given these criteria, practitioners may have appointments or selected clinical privileges denied or withdrawn, not because their practice is substandard in terms of traditional measures of quality but because it is economically inefficient (Hershey, 1994). For example, practice protocols are being developed within many organizations to increase cost efficiency. A failure to follow the protocols in the absence of a clinical contraindication could constitute an economic rationale for loss of privileges related to that particular case type or procedure.

It would be dangerous to use economic criteria exclusively in making appointment and privileging decisions. For example, withholding a procedure solely to bring the case in under the "dollar wire" of the DRG category when procedure performance would clearly constitute the standard of care would not support a quality outcome for the patient and could also be viewed as malpractice if patient harm resulted from the omission. Such emphasis on economy would be ethically unacceptable to all practitioners. Additionally, improper use of economic credentialing might constitute a restraint of trade (Blum, 1995). Using economic efficiency as an additional parameter when judging the professional and technical competence of an individual, however, may be inescapable within the current fiscal environment. We might even legitimately construe that increasing economic efficiency while maintaining equal or better quality is in the best interest of patients and the future survival of the health-care industry.

At present, economic credentialing is primarily aimed at physicians. As the numbers of practicing ACNPs increase, however, the same criteria will undoubtedly be applied to them as well. When ACNPs collaborate with physicians, the cost-efficiency measures for the combined services of the nurse and physician are melded. Cost inefficiency on the part of one partner affects the other. ACNPs may wish to investigate the economic efficiency of physicians with whom they are considering entering a collaborative relationship. Likewise, they should document their own economic effectiveness to demonstrate individual efficacy and cost savings to the organization and enhance their marketability.

Potential Pros and Cons of the Credentialing and Privileging Process for Acute Care Nurse Practitioners

The credentialing and privileging process may have both positive and negative implications for ACNP practice. Some may consider as a positive implication the notion that undergoing credentialing and privileging may serve to confer a sense of "increased legitimacy" of the ACNP in the eyes of patients and physicians. The state by state variation in scope of practice for NPs is frequently confusing to the public and potential physician collaborators. The nurse practice acts may be fairly nonspecific, and physicians who wish to collaborate with NPs may be uncomfortable with the "lack of details" regarding specificity of the actions that are within the scope of NP practice for that state. The lack of a requirement for a system for national (second) licensure, educational program certification, mandatory completion of the national certification examination, or mandatory continuing education is perceived by some to provide a "loose" system with little control of the quality of the NP product. In the eyes of these individuals, the credentialing and privileging process provides a mechanism for increased specificity and quality control. In addition, the process provides (at least theoretically) the opportunity for peer review, oversight, and self-governance.

Alternatively, the credentialing and privileging process may be viewed to place unnecessary restraints on the ACNPs scope of practice and efficacy. Restricting the ACNP from performing acts that they are educated and competent to perform, and sanctioned by law to execute, does not permit the full benefit and potential of the role to be realized. The potential for enhanced quality of patient care and system effectiveness afforded by ACNP practice would be undeveloped. It is also likely that extreme job dissatisfaction would result (the "H&P machine" syndrome). Additionally, restricting individuals from performing professional acts that they are licensed to provide may place a restraint on their trade and be viewed as antitrust activity. The review of situations and laws defining antitrust activity are beyond the scope of this chapter but are abundant in the literature (Grumet, 1993; Jacobsen & Wiggins, 1992; Kopit & Lutes, 1993; Roggensack, 1995; Timmons & Ridenour, 1993, 1994).

In the peer review process at the heart of the credentialing and privileging, questions of technical, professional, or personal misconduct of a professional are reviewed for departure from accepted standards, hopefully under due process. If the individual under review is found to have departed from accepted standards, limitation or termination of their privileges at the institution may be recommended, with clinical privilege restrictions of greater than 30 day's duration reported to the NPDB (Segall & Pearl, 1993). It is important that advanced practice nurses lead or are at least a part of this process. Review of an ACNPs activities that are conducted solely by other categories of providers would fail to provide peer perspective.

CONCLUSION

The ACNP role is being increasingly used in acute care organizations and systems. This chapter provides an overview of some of the organizational considerations related to ACNP practice. The organization newly using this role needs to increase its understanding of the role and take steps to ensure smooth assimilation of the practitioner into the system in order to achieve maximum benefits. Important considerations for system readiness include establishing the practice model and developing the organizational scope and standards of practice. Likewise, ACNPs must be aware of how they can structure their practice to meet organizational as well as patient care needs and be successful corporate members. Issues related to implementing the individual ACNP's practice include credentialing and privileging.

REFERENCES

American Nurses Association & American Association of Critical Care Nurses. (1995). *Standards of clinical practice and scope of practice for acute care nurse practitioner.* Washington, DC: American Nurses Publishing.

Ankney, R.N., Coil, J.A., Kolff, J., & Esper, E. (1995). Physician understanding of the national practitioner data bank. *Southern Medical Journal, 88*(2), 200–203.

Arthur v. St. Peter's Memorial Hospital, 169 N.J. Super. 575 (Laws Div. 1975).

Benesch, K. (1993). Medical staff privileges and "economic credentialing." *Trends in Health Care, Law & Ethics, 8*(4), 58–60.

Benesch, K. (1994). Emerging theories of liability for negligent credentialing in HMOs, integrated delivery and managed care systems. *Trends in Health Care, Law & Ethics, 9*(4), 41–46.

Birkholz, G. (1991). Implications of the national practitioner data bank for nurse practitioners. *Health Care Issues, 16*(8), 40–46.

Birkholz, G. (1995). Malpractice data from the national practitioner data bank. *Nurse Practitioner, 20* (3), 32–35.

Blum, J.D. (1995). Economic credentialing moves from the hospital to managed care. *J Health Care Finance, 22*(1), 60–71.

Brandt, M. (1996). Frequently asked questions on joint commission standards. *Journal of AHIMA, 67*(5), 34–37.

Burkholder, J.S., & Dudjak, L.A. (1994). The midlevel practitioner role: One medical center's experience. *AACN Clinical Issues, 5*(3), 369–403.

Corleto v. Shore Memorial Hospital, 138 N.J. Super. 302, 350 A.2d 534 (1975).

Culbertson, R.A. (1991). National practitioner data bank has implications for nursing. *Nursing Outlook, 39*(3), 102–103, 142.

Darling v. Charleston Memorial Hospital, 33III.2d326;211 N.E. 2d 253 (1965), cert. denied 383 U.S. 946 (1966).

Dent, T.L. (1996). Training and privileging for new procedures. *Surgical Clinics of North America, 76*(3), 615–621.

Dracup, K., DeBusk, R.F., DeMoyts, H., Gaile, E.H., Norton, J.B., & Rudy, E.B. (1994). Task Force 3; Partnership in delivery of cardiovascular care. *American Journal of Critical Care, 24,* 296–303.

Eliason, B.C. (1994). More on the privileging process. *Family Medicine, 26*(4), 206.

Ferguson v. Gonyaw, 64 Mich. App. 685, 235 N.W. 2d 543 (1976).

Ford, L. (1997). A voice from the past: 30 fascinating years as a nurse practitioner. *Clinical Excellence for Nurse Practitioners, 1*(1), 3–6.

Gabel, W.K. (1993). National practitioner data bank. *Journal of the American Optometric Association, 64* (2), 133–135.

Gilliam, J. W. II. (1994). A contemporary analysis of medicolegal concerns for physician assistants and nurse practitioners. In C.H. Wecht (Ed.), *Legal medicine 1994* (pp. 133–180). Salem, NH: Butterworth Legal Publishers.

Grumet, B.R. (1993). Current and emerging legal issues in critical care. *Critical Care Clinics, 9*(3), 465–476.

Hall, J.K. (1993). How to analyze nurse practitioner licensure laws. *Nurse Practitioner, 18*(8), 31–34.

Harty-Golder, B. (Ed.). (1993). Applying for medical staff membership. Peer review part I. *J. Florida M.A., 80*(6), 413–415.

Hershey, N. (1994). Economic credentialing: A poor title for a legitimate assessment concept. *American Journal of Medical Quality, 9*(1), 3–9.

Hravnak, M., & Baldisseri M. (1997). Credentialing and privileging: Insight into the process. *AACN Clinical Issues, 8,* 108–115.

Hravnak, M., & Magdic, K. (1997). Marketing the acute care nurse practitioner. *Clinical Excellence for Nurse Practitioners, 1*(1), 9–13.

Hravnak, M., Rosenzweig, M.Q., & Baldisseri, M. (1996). Current questions with regard to acute care nurse practitioners preparation and role implementation. *AACN Clinical Issues, 7*(2), 289–299.

Hudson, T. (1993). Factoring in the financials: Court gives nod to economic credentialing. *Hospitals, 67*(7), 36–40.

Jacobsen, R. A. Jr., & Wiggins, R.B. (1992). Denial of staff privileges fact increased antitrust scrutiny. *Health Care Management Review, 17*(4), 7–15.

Johnson v. Misericordia Community Hospital, 99 Wis, 2d 708, 301 N.W. 2d 156 (1981).

Kolb, D.S., Hughes, R.L., & Young, C.E. (1993). Economic credentialing. *Topics in Health Care Financing, 19*(3), 58–66.

Kopit, W.G., & Lutes, M.E. (1993). Legal issues and antitrust considerations in the establishment of credentialing and other selection criteria. In. P.R. Kongsvedt (Ed.), *The managed health care handbook* (pp. 461–480). Gaithersburg, MD: Aspen Publishers.

Kristeller, A. R. (1995). Medical staff: Privileging and credentialing. *New Jersey Medicine, 92*(1), 26–28.

Mitchell v. Joiner, 229 Ga. 140, 189 S.E.2d 412 (1971).

Musallam, L.S. (1995). Privileges, credentialing, and liability. *Primary Care: Clinics in Office Practice, 22*(3), 491–498.

Norris, T.E., & Susman, J. L. (1995). Bringing science and rationality to privileging and credentialing issues. *American Family Physician, 52*(3), 785–490.

Parinello, K.M. (1995). Advanced practice nursing: An administrative perspective. *Critical Care Nursing Clinics of North America, 7*(1), 9–16.

Pearson, L.G. (1995). Annual updates of how each state stands on legislative issues affecting advanced nursing practice. *Nursing Practice, 20,* 13–51.

Pearson, L.G. (1996). Annual updates of how each state stands on legislative issues affecting advanced nursing practice. *Nursing Practice, 21,* 10–70.

Pearson, L.G. (1997). Annual updates of how each state stands on legislative issues affecting advanced nursing practice. *Nursing Practice, 22,* 18–82.

Price, T.E. (1993). Economic credentialing revisited: Watch out, here it comes! *Journal of Medical Association of Georgia, 82,* 21–23.

Purcell v. Zimbelman, 18 Ariz. App. 75, 500 P.2d 335 (1972).

Richmond, T., & Keane, A. (1996). Acute care nurse practitioners. In H.V. Hickey, R.M. Ouimette & S.L. Venegoni (Eds.), *Advance practice nursing: Changing roles and clinical applications.* Philadelphia: Lippincott.

Roggensack, P.D. (1995). Medical staff bylaws are violated by hospital's ICU restrictions. *Wisconsin Medical Journal, 94*(11), 631–632.

Segall, S.E., & Pearl, W. (1993). Should due process be part of hospital peer review [Editorial]? *Southern Medical Journal, 86(*3), 368–369.

Shala, T. (1991). Changing regulator environment requires stronger risk management controls. *Journal of AMRA, 62*(2), 34–38.

Smith, A.C. (1993). Obtaining hospitals privileges for advanced practice nurse. *Journal of Pediatric Health Care, 7,* 292–293.

Smith, T.C. (1991). A structured process to credential nurses with advanced practice skills. *Journal of Nursing Quality Assurance, 5*(3), 40–51.

Spisso, J., O'Callaghan, C., McKennan, M., & Holcroft, J.W. (1990). Improved quality of care and reduction of house staff workload using trauma nurse practitioners. *Journal of Trauma, 30,* 660–665.

Stahl, D.A. (1995). Managed care credentialing. *Nursing Management, 26*(6), 18,20.

Susman, J. & Rodney, W.M. (1994). Editorial: Numbers, procedural skills and science: Do the three mix [Editorial]? *American Family Physician, 49*(7), 1591–1592.

Timmons, G., & Ridenour N. (1993). Restraint of trade implications for nurse practitioners: Denial of hospital admitting or staff privileges. *Journal of the American Academy of Nurse Practitioners, 5*(4), 175–178.

Timmons, G., & Ridenour, N. (1994). Legal approaches to the restraint of trade of nurse practitioners: Disparate reimbursement patterns. *Journal of the American Academy of Nurse Practitioners, 6*(2), 55–59.

5

Collaboration: The Essence of Acute Care Nurse Practitioner Practice

Kathleen B. King and Judith G. Baggs*

Although the words *advanced practice nursing* are relatively new, nurses in advanced clinical practice have been around for at least half a century. Reiter (1966) wrote about the efficacy of nurse-clinicians in enhancing the care of people admitted to hospitals, stating that the role for nurses with advanced clinical ability was begun in 1943. Grounded in a community health background, Ford and Silver (1967) formulated the nurse practitioner role in the provision of primary care to children. Although not without debate, both of these efforts were innovative and fostered an environment of creative change in nursing (Bigbee, 1996). Over the past few years what had become the traditional categorization of advanced practice nurses into clinical nurse specialists (acute or specialty care) and nurse practitioners (primary care) is increasingly seen as arbitrary as the recognition of a variety of roles for nurses in advanced practice emerges. Indeed, in the acute care arena, titles have appeared in an attempt to capture developing roles and responsibilities, such as acute care nurse practitioner (Davitt & Jensen, 1981) and tertiary nurse practitioner (Keane & Richmond, 1993). Some argue for maintaining the traditional distinctions between clinical nurse

*The first author would like to acknowledge the advice of her 9-year-old daughter, Genevieve King Laing. "Just get to the point mom—say that nurses and doctors are equal."

specialists and nurse practitioners (Page & Arena, 1994). Health care delivery is changing, however, and just as innovators before us advocated for changing and expanding the roles nurses play in the delivery of care, nursing would be wise to do the same today.

What is interesting is that although appropriate roles have been debated, the idea of collaboration has permeated the advanced practice literature, whether in papers referring to clinical nurse specialists or in those concerning nurse practitioners. Collaboration with patients and families is taken as fundamental for all advanced practice nurses, yet differences in the professional targets of collaboration are apparent, depending on the body of literature one reads. The clinical nurse specialist literature tends to focus on collaboration with other nurses (e.g., staff nurses, nurse educators, nurse researchers, nurse administrators) and, to a lesser extent, other health care providers. The nurse practitioner literature (including the newly emerging acute care nurse practitioner literature) tends to focus on collaboration with physicians. We believe that collaboration among all providers is necessary for success of advanced practice nurses in acute care. When all forms of collaboration are developed and fostered, practice is more informed and the opportunity to improve care is maximized. Thus, we will attempt to address the full range of collaborative practice in this chapter.

DEFINITION OF COLLABORATIVE PRACTICE

In its broadest sense collaboration is defined as working together. This definition can be applied to many types of endeavors and becomes most useful when the goals of collaboration are specified. In the clinical setting collaboration is providers "cooperatively working together, sharing responsibility for solving problems and making decisions to formulate and carry out plans for patient care" (Baggs & Schmitt, 1988, p. 145). For collaboration to be fully realized, the collaborative partners should be part of a stable team, although the mix of providers constituting a team varies across differing practice sites or patient populations. Much of what has been written about collaboration focuses on interactions between staff nurses and physicians, often resident physicians, and is covered in other reviews (Baggs & Schmitt, 1988).

Central to a collaborative practice model is that patient needs are the foremost priority in the provision of care (Chavigny, 1993; DeAngelis, 1994). Emphasis is on patient outcomes. In order to effect quality outcomes, professionals assume responsibility in the provision of care for which they are best prepared. In acute care, a collaborative practice model is based on the idea that the patients require the services of different types of providers simultaneously for each encounter or hospital admission (King, Parrinello, & Baggs, 1995). Different types of providers, including but not limited to advanced practice nurses, staff nurses, and physicians, make unique contributions in affecting the outcome of each patient's problem. This assumes that for a significant number of functions, one type of provider cannot substitute for another member of the team. Some functions may be performed by more than one type of provider, but more cannot. If one provider substitutes for another and tries to provide for the unique functions of another, the best outcome may not be achieved. An example of unique functions would be that the surgeon has primary authority and responsibility for the patient in the operating room, whereas the advanced practice nurse has primary authority and responsibility regarding patient teaching, discharge planning, and the decision to discharge the patient (Norsen, Opladen, & Quinn, 1995). Collaboration in this context is viewed as interdependent interdisciplinary practice and adheres to the belief that optimal patient outcomes cannot be obtained by a solitary provider but require the abilities and expertise of a variety of members of the collaborative team (Norsen et al., 1995; Pike, McHugh, & Canney, 1993).

COLLABORATIVE PRACTICE AND THE ADVANCED PRACTICE NURSE

Collaboration between the advanced practice nurse and other nurses has been addressed fairly extensively within the traditional delineation of the functions of the clinical nurse specialist (American Nurses Association, 1980). These functions include practice, consultation, education, and research in which the advanced practice nurse or clinical nurse specialist collaborates with other providers largely through indirect care activities (Walton, Jakobowski, & Barnsteiner, 1993). Relative to the practice function, the clinical nurse specialist often is administratively responsible to nursing practice and plays a major role in supporting the nursing staff through the formulation of nursing plans of care for specialty groups of patients. In addition, collaboration with physicians has been viewed within the context of carrying out the medical plan. "The clinical nurse specialist is able to influence nursing practice so that medical regimens are consistently carried out according to the requirements of the patient population" (Walton et al., 1993, p. 58). Thus, the coordination of nursing and medical care plans for a specialty population has been recognized as a hallmark for advanced nursing practice in acute care, and the road to achieving coordinated care is often placed in the context of collaboration with all types of providers.

Increasingly, attention has focused on collaborative practice involving the advanced practice nurse and the physician in acute care, with the extension of the advanced practice nurse role beyond provision of indirect care. Some advocate that the advanced practice nurse–physician dyad forms the core of collaborative practice in the acute care setting (Genet et al., 1995; Norsen et al., 1995). Establishing a collaborative practice in which the advanced practice nurse and attending physician compose the core team has the advantage of providing for ongoing continuity and coordination of care (Davitt & Jensen, 1981; Norsen et al., 1995). Although the dyad is seen as core, the advanced practice nurse is viewed as a sophisticated practitioner who integrates responsibilities for direct patient care with indirect activities such as consultation, research and leadership. Such integration is necessary to complement the focus and goals of collaboration (Norsen et al., 1995). This approach exemplifies the use of direct and indirect patient care skills within the advanced practice role in acute care.

In formulating the collaborative dyad between advanced practice nurses and physicians, a critical assumption is that the core collaborative practice team comprises advanced practice nurses and physicians who have attained full professional status (Gleeson et al., 1990; Norsen et al., 1995). Each partner will have completed her or his basic education and postgraduate training, thus the core collaborative team comprises the advanced practice nurse and the attending physician. This element is essential in order for a collaborative practice team to take advantage of and use the full scope of practice of each of the partners.

This assumption speaks against the resident replacement model that has been advocated by some as a role for advanced practice nurses. Using advanced practice nurses to substitute for a medical or surgical resident has several disadvantages. One disadvantage is that the advanced practice nurse's scope of practice is defined only as that part that is a subset of the attending physician's scope. The full scope of advanced practice nursing is not recognized, in that those functions unique to the nurse practitioner are truncated. In addition, the advanced practice nurse is put in the position of being supervised by the attending physician and is equated with a trainee, rather than being viewed as a true complementary partner.

At the same time, it is important to understand the opportunity provided for advanced practice nurses in the acute care setting, where trainee positions in specialty care are being reduced or threatened to be reduced. This trend has motivated many physicians and administrators to recognize, some for the first time, areas of overlap between physician practice and advanced nursing practice. Advanced practice nurses can capitalize on this recognition in settings where the number of trainees are being reduced. It is imperative, however, to appreciate the areas of advanced nursing practice that are unique and independently contribute to desired patient outcomes. Failing to recognize the full scope of advanced nursing practice has the potential to promote undervaluing of their contributions in the long run.

SUPPORT FOR COLLABORATIVE PRACTICE

Since the early 1980s a number of publications from national organizations have supported collaborative care, although the emphasis on collaborative practice for advanced practice nurses was not specified. One of the earliest was the American Nurses Association's *Nursing: A Social Policy Statement* (1980). In 1982 the American Association of Critical Care Nurses and the Society for Critical Care Medicine published guidelines in support of collaborative practice in critical care units. The Institute of Medicine (1983), the National Commission on Nursing (1981), and the Secretary's Commission on Nursing (1988) all produced documents that were supportive of collaborative care.

In addition to beliefs about the importance of collaboration there is a research literature that has consistently found associations between collaborative care and improved patient outcomes. The first evidence came from the work of the National Joint Practice Commission (NJPC) in the early 1970s. The NJPC was a group composed of equal numbers of physicians and nurses and was founded by the American Medical Association and the American Nurses Association in 1971 to recommend ways for physicians and nurses to improve the quality of health care delivery by working together (NJPC, 1981).

The importance of collaborative practice for advanced practice nurses has been stressed by many leaders and pioneers in nursing. Kitzman (1986) wrote of collaboration between advanced practice nurses and physicians as a way to organize a practice to enhance quality of care and improve patient outcomes.

On the other hand, the importance of collaboration between nurses and physicians has been less clearly presented in the medical literature. As several nonnurse commentators have noted, discussions of the relationships between nurses and physicians are found primarily in nursing journals, whereas physicians have seldom written on this topic (McMahan, Hoffman, & McGee, 1994). In the preceding statement the authors were speaking of any discussion of interactions, not just of discussions of collaboration.

Where physicians have written about collaboration, they have generally been positive. Stein (1967) wrote about the "doctor-nurse game," a communication model that requires the nurse to convince physicians that any recommendations made were instigated by the physician, even when the idea was the nurse's. This mode of communication was designed to obtain the best possible care for the patient while saving face for physicians who believed they should initiate any changes in care. Stein saw it as interfering with good care, however. McMahan and colleagues (1994) wrote of the historical background to this behavior. They said, "physician-nurse relationships are mired in an ideology as old as medicine itself; it is an ideology that exacerbates role conflicts and that permits the continued perceptions of inequalities and lack of collaboration between the two professions" (p. 91). Bates (1966) spoke of differences in what was valued by nurses and physicians. For example, physicians assessed nurses positively for assisting skillfully, following orders, and deviating from policies. On the other hand, nurses assessed physicians positively for conserving nursing resources and honoring policies. Bates believed that these differences created difficulties in developing care together but that shared decision making leading to better care could be facilitated when both providers focus on the common goal of what is needed for the patient's welfare (Bates, 1970). More recently, Stein, Watts, and Howell (1990) updated Stein's earlier work (1967), writing positively about a new lack of hierarchy, a more open and collegial relationship, which they believe fosters better patient care.

A few papers have supported the efficacy of collaborative practice between advanced practice nurses in acute care and physicians, although all are written from the nursing perspective and most are anecdotal. The first collaborative practice effort between an acute care nurse practitioner and a group of surgeons was begun in 1979 in cardiothoracic surgery at the University of Rochester Medical Center (Davitt & Jensen, 1981). More recently, the role of nurse practitioners in acute care has been described in a medical patient care division (Genet et al., 1995) and a head and neck surgical oncology practice (Martin & Coniglio, 1996). In a recent phenomenological study, Arslanian-Engoren (1995) examined the perspective of clinical nurse specialists and their collaborative practices with physicians. Five themes emerged: mutual trust and respect, maintaining a nursing perspective, establishing collegial relationships, defining a practice role, and living a positive experience. Collaboration was seen as a satisfying experience in which the nurses could accomplish the goals of advanced practice nursing. Although collaboration between advanced practice nurses and physicians were addressed in each of these papers, they also addressed the collaborative role of advanced practice nurses with other health care providers, especially staff nurses. All of these papers support a collaborative practice model for enhancing patient care that merges both direct and indirect care responsibilities for the advanced practice nurse.

BARRIERS TO COLLABORATIVE PRACTICE

Barriers to collaboration arise from both nurses and physicians. On the physician side, organized medicine has traditionally seen itself as owning the entire domain of health care. Unfortunately, nurses also can play into this view. For example, nurses have debated about whether advanced practice nurses are "mini-doctors" selling out to the medical model. This argument inadvertently supports the notion that medicine "owns" much of health care and that physicians retain the right to apportion parts of care or tasks to fit their needs. The claim that nurses were "practicing medicine" was made about the early pediatric and primary care nurse practitioner roles because those practitioners performed functions that up until that point had been done only by physicians. This same message can be heard today regarding acute care nurse practitioners. Is the problem that nurses are "acting like doctors?" Or is the issue the fact that organized medicine has staked out all of health care as its own, parceling out only those pieces that physicians do not have the inclination (or training) to do, all the time claiming that they really could do it all if they only had the time. There is a growing recognition that physicians do not own it all and that other providers can effectively deliver a wider and more comprehensive range of care than the traditional hierarchial model suggests.

On an individual level, nurses may be threatened by the increased responsibility and accountability involved in collaborative practice (Cape, 1986; Prescott, Dennis, & Jacox, 1987). For nurses to collaborate they need to be willing to assume accountability and increased authority in practice areas. It is much easier to sit back and critique someone else's decisions than to have responsibility for making those decisions. For example, an advanced practice nurse who always defers to a physician in making patient care decisions is free to "Monday morning quarterback" the decisions made and critique them in light of any negative outcomes. This behavior is not collaborative but dependent and leads to delayed decision making and delayed patient care.

No studies were found that examined collaboration between acute care nurse practitioners and physicians. Lamb and Napodano (1984), however, found little collaboration between advanced practice nurses and the physicians with whom they worked in primary care. They defined collaboration as requiring face-to-face communication, contributions from each provider, and integration of ideas to formulate a new solution. Only 23% of the taped interactions between the advanced practice nurse and the physician qualified as collaborative (Lamb & Napodano, 1984). McLain (1988a, 1988b) studied primary care teams and found both physicians and nurses were contributors to conditions blocking collaborative care. Both physicians and nurse practitioners engaged in distorted communication and nonmeaningful interactions that blocked collaborative practice (McLain, 1988a, 1988b). She concluded that there are few empirical data to support the actual existence of collaborative practice as a predominant pattern between nurses and physicians.

Another barrier to collaboration between nurses and physicians has been the perceived differences in educational preparation and skills between the two groups (Stichler, 1995). Prescott and Bowen (1985) found that competence of physicians was assumed by both physicians and nurses but that nurses had to prove their competence in each interaction, in part because how the nurses were educated was very different, whereas medical education was more standardized. Stichler (1995) noted that the higher level education of advanced practice nurses, "their demonstrated competency and advanced clinical knowledge contributes to the development of nurse-physician collaborative practice" (p. 58).

ELEMENTS OF COLLABORATION IN ADVANCED PRACTICE

Baggs (1994) defined six critical elements that describe the substance of collaborative practice: cooperation, assertiveness, shared decisionmaking, communication, planning together, and coordination. Trust is the glue that synthesizes these elements to optimize the goals of collaborative practice (Miccolo & Spanier, 1993). When trust is the foundation for the collaborative relationships, cooperation can exist, assertiveness does not become threatening, shared decision-making is not avoided, communication is not hampered, and coordination is not haphazard (Norsen et al., 1995). Others also have identified mutual trust and respect as a basic theme for collaboration between advanced practice nurses and physicians (Arslanian-Engoren, 1995; King, 1990). Mutual trust and respect among the advanced practice nurse, staff nurses, and nurse managers is equally essential for the delivery of excellent patient-centered care to be achieved. This trust is not limited to direct patient care activities but also encompasses the advanced practice nurse's expertise in indirect patient care activities through consultation, education, and research. The indirect care functions of the advanced practice role cannot be overemphasized. Evidence-based practice has become the standard by which care is measured. The advanced practice nurse can play a significant role in using the most up-to-date evidence (i.e., data-based research) to inform nursing and medical care. In addition, the advanced practice nurse is in an optimal position to help generate data through research activities that can inform patient care in the future.

Davitt and Jensen (1981) described coordination of care and continuity and consistency in provision of care as elements that formed the foundation for the acute care nurse practitioner role. These elements are played out in an interdisciplinary approach as the acute care nurse practitioner collaborates with nursing and medical staff to develop, implement, and evaluate each patient's plan of care. As well, standards of care are collaboratively formulated for groups of patients.

Coordination of care is a priority activity for the nurse practitioner in acute care. Coordination of nursing and medical care has the advantage of reducing redundancy and duplication of assessment and management of patients (Genet et al., 1995). Complete elimination of redundancy in the initial assessment of patients should not be a goal. First, repeating a history and physical examination may jog a patient's or a family's memory and thus better inform the plan of care. Second, extreme biological variations, for example blood pressure readings, often revert to less extreme values on repeated examination, enabling a more informed decision regarding a plan of action. Lastly, a repeated examination may simply uncover information that was previously missed (Sackett, Haynes, Guyatt, & Tugwell, 1991). Ongoing assessment of patients in the critical and acute care environments is a standard of care; redundancy of assessments by multiple providers, however, can be held to a minimum through the coordination of care by the advanced practice nurse. Elimination of redundancy of care management can be a goal once the plan of care is formulated in collaborative interactions.

Continuity and consistency in provision of care is optimally achieved when the advanced practice nurse and attending physician form the core of the collaborative team. Both participants in this dyad are permanent members of the team, allowing for stability and continuity. Both participate in the long-term evaluation of the care delivered to the group of patients, both ensure that the standard of patient care is of high quality, and both participate in the education of trainees in nursing and medicine (Davitt & Jensen, 1981).

SUMMARY

Collaboration is the future for all health care providers and is particularly the essence of practice for the advanced practice nurse in acute care. It replaces the traditional turf protectionism that can undermine patient-centered care. Collaboration reduces redundancy, enhances continuity, and works toward the elimination of fragmentation in the delivery of care to acutely ill people. The advanced practice nurse can be viewed as keeping the patient as the focal point through collaborative practice in the acute care environment.

REFERENCES

American Association of Critical Care Nurses. (1982). *Collaborative practice model: The organization of human resources in critical care units.* Newport Beach, CA: Author.

American Nurses Association. (1980). *Nursing: A social policy statement.* Kansas City, MO: Author.

Arslanian-Engoren, C. M. (1995). Lived experience of CNSs who collaborate with physicians: A phenomenological study. *Clinical Nurse Specialist, 9,* 68–74.

Baggs, J.G. (1994). Development of an instrument to measure collaboration and satisfaction about care decisions. *Journal of Advanced Nursing, 20,* 176–182.

Baggs, J. G., & Schmitt, M. H. (1988). Collaboration between nurses and physicians. *Image: Journal of Nursing Scholarship, 20,* 145–149.

Bates, B. (1966). Nurse-physician teamwork. *Medical Care, 4,* 69–80.

Bates, B. (1970). Doctor and nurse: Changing roles and relations. *New England Journal of Medicine, 283,* 129–134.

Bigbee, J.L. (1996). History and evolution of advanced practice nursing. In A.B. Hamric, J.A. Spross, & C.M. Hanson (Eds.), *Advanced nursing practice: An integrative approach* (pp. 3–24). Philadelphia: W.B. Saunders.

Cape, L.S. (1986). Collaborative practice models and structures. In D.A. England (Ed.), *Collaboration in nursing* (pp. 13–26). Rockville, MD: Aspen.

Chavigny, K. H. (1993). AMA's policies and nursing's role in emerging systems. *Nursing Management, 24,* 30–34.

Davitt, P. A., & Jensen, L. A. (Fall, 1981). The role of the acute care nurse practitioner in cardiac surgery. *Nursing Administration Quarterly,* 16–19.

DeAngelis, C. D. (1994). Nurse practitioner redux. *Journal of the American Medical Association, 271,* 868–871.

Ford, L. C., & Silver, H. K. (1967). The expanded role of the nurse in child care. *Nursing Outlook, 15,* 43–45.

Genet, C. A., Brennan, P. F., Ibbotson-Wolff, S., et al. (1995). Nurse practitioners in a teaching hospital. *Nurse Practitioner, 20,* 47–54.

Gleeson, R. M., McIlvain-Simpson, G., Boos, M. L., Sweet, E., Trzcinski, K. M., Solberg, C. A., & Doughty, R. A. (1990). Advanced practice nursing: A model of collaborative care. *Maternal Child Nursing, 15,* 9–12.

Institute of Medicine. (1983). *Nursing and nursing education.* Washington DC: National Academy Press.

Keane, A., & Richmond, T. (1993). Tertiary nurse practitioners. *Image, 25,* 281–284.

King, M. B. (1990). Clinical nurse specialist collaboration with physicians. *Clinical Nurse Specialist, 4,* 172–177.

King, K. B., Parrinello, K. A., & Baggs, J. G. (1995). Collaboration and advanced practice nursing. In J. V. Hickey, R. M. Ouimette, & S.L. Venegoni (Eds.), *Advanced practice nursing: Changing roles and clinical applications* (pp. 146 162). Philadelphia: Lippincott.

Kitzman, H. (1986). Education in nursing. In J. E. Steel (Ed.) *Issues in collaborative practice* (pp.139–159). Orlando: Grune & Stratton.

Lamb, G. S., & Napodano, R. J. (1984). Physician-nurse practitioner interaction patterns in primary care practices. *American Journal of Public Health, 74,* 26–29.

Martin, B. & Coniglio, J.U. (1996). The acute care nurse practioner in collaborative practice. *AACN Clinical Issues, 7,* 309–314.

McLain, B. R. (1988a). Collaborative practice: The nurse practitioner's role in its success or failure. *Nurse Practitioner, 13,* 31–38.

McLain, B. R. (1988b). Collaborative practice: A critical theory perspective. *Research in Nursing and Health, 11,* 391–398.

McMahan, E. M., Hoffman, K., & McGee, G. W. (1994). Physician-nurse relationships in clinical settings: A review and critique of the literature, 1966–1992. *Medical Care Review, 51,* 83–112.

Miccolo, M., & Spanier, A. (1993). Critical care management in the 1990s: Making collaborative practice work. *Critical Care Clinics, 9,* 443–453.

National Commission on Nursing. (1981). *Initial report and preliminary recommendations.* Chicago: American Hospital Association.

National Joint Practice Commission (NJPC). (1981). *Guidelines for establishing joint or collaborative practice in hospitals.* Chicago: Author.

Norsen, L., Opladen, J., & Quinn, J. (1995). Practice model: Collaborative practice. *Critical Care Nursing Clinics of North America, 7,* 43–52.

Page, N.E., & Arena, D.M. (1994). Rethinking the merger of the clinical nurse specialist and the nurse practitioner roles. *Image, 26,* 315–318.

Pike, A. W., McHugh, M., & Canney, K. (1993). A new architecture for quality assurance: Nurse physician collaboration. *Journal of Nursing Care Quality, 7,* 1–8.

Prescott, P. A., & Bowen, S. A. (1985). Physician-nurse relationships. *Annals of Internal Medicine, 103,* 127–133.

Prescott, P. A., Dennis, K. E., & Jacox, A. K. (1987). Clinical decision making of staff nurses. *Image, 19,* 56–62.

Reiter F. (1966). The nurse-clinician. *American Journal of Nursing, 66,* 274–80.

Sackett, D.L., Haynes, R.B., Guyatt, G.H., & Tugwell, P. (1991). *Clinical epidemiology* (2nd ed.). Boston: Little Brown.

Secretary's Commission on Nursing. (1988). *Final report* (Vol. I). Washington, DC: Department of Health and Human Services.

Stein, L. I. (1967). The doctor-nurse game. *Archives of General Psychiatry, 16,* 699–703.

Stein, L. I., Watts, D. T., & Howell, T. (1990). The doctor-nurse game revisited. *New England Journal of Medicine, 322,* 546–549.

Stichler, J.F. (1995). Professional interdependence: The art of collaboration. *Advanced Practice Nursing Quarterly, 1,* 53–61.

Walton, M. K., Jakobowski, D. S., & Barnsteiner, J. H. (1993). A collaborative practice model for the clinical nurse specialist. *Journal of Nursing Administration, 23,* 55–59.

6

Negotiating Skills: Empowering the Acute Care Nurse Practitioner

JoAnne Herman, Amelia K. Selph, Marguerite L. Knox, Janet S. Nussbaum, and Rachel Franklin

Acute care nurse practitioners (ACNPs) are a relatively new addition to the health-care team. Programs that prepare ACNPs and job opportunities for these graduates have flourished in the mid-1990s (Clochesy, Daly, Idemoto, Steel, & Fitzpatrick, 1994). Because the role is evolving simultaneously with the redesign of the American health-care system, ACNPs are confronted with a great deal of ambiguity and instability in the system (Hadley, 1996). ACNPs are pioneers blazing the trail in this new and exciting territory that contains both great opportunities and major obstacles. In this environment, communicating value and worth of ACNPs to potential consumers of services, defining role characteristics and boundaries, negotiating perquisites and benefits, and establishing the relative balance of power within an employment situation are essential. The purpose of this chapter is to describe strategies for negotiating this new territory. Specifically, we will explore the process of negotiation, describe portfolio development, discuss the contractual issues of negotiating with an individual or practice group, and suggest methods for dealing with resistance to the role.

NEGOTIATING

The following section introduces the concept of negotiation, describes the elements in the process, and identifies some specific strategies that ACNPs can use to increase the power of their negotiating position. Donaldson and Donaldson (1996) define a negotiation as "any communication in which you are attempting to achieve the approval, acquiescence, or action of someone else (p.1)." They divide the negotiating process into six elements: preparing, setting limits and goals, managing emotions, listening, communicating clearly, and closing the deal. ACNPs can be much more successful in negotiating by being aware of the elements of the process and improving skills in each element.

All negotiations should start with an understanding of the outcome to be accomplished. In this case, the outcome is a personally, professionally, and financially fulfilling position as an ACNP. That position may be different for every person depending on his or her personal desires for life. Your task is to determine the specifics for your situation.

Preparation for the Negotiation

Knowledge is power in any negotiating situation. The more knowledge you have about yourself and the situation, the more powerful your negotiating position will be. Preparation begins with a thorough and honest self-evaluation. This process is like corporate strategic planning. You are developing the trajectory for your life over the next few years. Start by establishing your goal. Then assess your strengths and weaknesses, personal and professional values, personal financial situation, salary and benefit requirements, professional development needs, and work environment requirements. The Personal Assessment Worksheet (Table 6.1) contains a list of specific questions to ask yourself. Spend time reflecting on each question, write down thorough answers, analyze your responses, and use your analysis to create your negotiating position.

Now that you have a clear understanding of who you are and what you need to be fulfilled in your professional life, obtain detailed information about the local marketplace and the characteristics of the practice with which you will be negotiating. The Marketplace Characteristics Worksheet (Table 6.2) contains key questions that you must answer in order to assess the marketplace and political climate in your area. The local marketplace includes state laws and regulations governing advanced practice, supply and demand for ACNPs, financial packages and scope of

TABLE 6.1 Personal Assessment Worksheet

GOALS

What are my 1-year goals?
  Personal:
  Professional:
What are my 5-year goals?
  Personal:
  Professional:

VALUES

What do I value personally?
What do I value professionally?

STRENGTHS/WEAKNESSES

What are my strengths?
What are my weaknesses?

FINANCIAL SITUATION

What salary do I want?
What salary do I require?
Am I willing to be paid based on productivity?

BENEFITS

What benefits do I need?
  Medical insurance?
  Family coverage?
  Dental insurance?
  Disability insurance?
  Life insurance?
  Retirement?
  Day care/medical reimbursement?
What benefits do I currently have that I will not need?
What benefits do I currently have that I need to continue?

TIME COMMITMENT

What hours do I want to work?
What time can I begin work?
What time do I need to leave work?
Am I willing to work weekends?
How much vacation time do I need?
Am I willing/able to work each day until the work is done?
Am I willing/able to take call?
  Weekend call?
  Week night call?

PROFESSIONAL DEVELOPMENT

What type of orientation do I want?
What type of mentoring do I expect?
How much autonomy am I willing to exercise?
How much continuing education (CE) do I need each year?

Continued

TABLE 6.1 *Continued*

How much does CE credit in my area cost?
What professional journals do I subscribe to?
  What are the costs?
What organizations am I a member of?
  What are the costs?
What are the professional expenses associated with my licensure/certification?
Prescriptive authority?
DEA #?
Yearly licensure?
Recertification?
Liability insurance?

WORK ENVIRONMENT
Will I need an office?
Will need a beeper or cellular phone?
Will I need additional support staff to complete my duties?
What computer or other equipment needs will I have?
What type of clients do I want to work with?
What age groups am I able to work with?
Can I do outpatient management?
Can I do inpatient management?
Am I interested in specialty or general practice?

practice for ACNPs in the area, and major competitors (Hupcey, 1993; Wilken, 1995).

Be aware that competition varies depending on location. It may be physicians, physician assistants, or nurse practitioners. In many instances, your biggest competitor is the prevailing attitude about advanced practice nurses. Identifying the role characteristics that make the ACNP a better candidate for an available position can give the ACNP the competitive edge. Think strategically about what information you want to highlight during the application and interview process. If you are competing against a physician or physician assistant, you want to emphasize ACNP scope of practice as well as the unique attributes of nurses, such as effective interpersonal skills, knowledge of teaching and learning principals, understanding of family dynamics, and resource use through case management. When other nurse practitioners are your competition, you want to highlight your past experiences and expertise. What knowledge and skills do you have that will set you apart from the others? The competition hardest to overcome is a negative attitude toward nurse practitioners. In a later section, we address strategies for dealing with resistance to the role.

The characteristics of the practice include typical clientele, services provided, payment mechanisms, provider mix, organizational structure, powerful people, reason for negotiating with an ACNP, and strengths and weaknesses of the practice. The Practice Characteristics Worksheet in Table 6.3 lists the

TABLE 6.2 Marketplace Assessment Worksheet

LAWS & REGULATIONS

What are the state laws governing my practice?
Do I have an copy for myself and my potential employer?
Are there any laws or regulations pending that will affect my practice?
Do I have up-to-date information on their progress and impact?

ACNP UTILIZATION

Are there other ACNPs in practice in my area?
Have I contacted them?
Have my potential employers ever employed an ACNP or other NP?
What was the outcome of that association?
What is the current job market for advanced practice nurses in my area?
What is the average salary and benefits package for persons in positions similar to the one I am seeking?

COMPETITION

Who are my major competitors?
Other ACNPs?
Other NPs?
Physician's assistants?
What are the role characteristics that make me a better candidate for this position?

FACILITY ISSUES

Does the facility I will be practicing in credential advanced practice nurses?
Are mechanisms in place for seeking privileges?
What are the limitations or barriers in the facility?

SCOPE OF PRACTICE

Do I have a copy of the Scope and Standards of Practice for the Acute Care Nurse Practitioners?
Do I have a copy of this document for my potential employer?
What is the scope of practice for persons in similar positions?
What are the usual job responsibilities for persons in similar positions?

POLITICS

What are the political issues surrounding advanced practice nurses in my area?
In my state?
Are their organizations or groups that I can use for support in my new role?
Who are the policy makers that I need to be in contact with?

TABLE 6.3 Practice Assessment Worksheet

CLIENTELE & SERVICES PROVIDED

What type of client is most often seen?
  Age groups?
What are the most common diagnoses managed?
What is the average inpatient census?
What is the average number of clients seen per day?
What is the average number of consultations or admissions per day?
Is this a specialty based practice?
Is this a consultation based practice?
What procedures are commonly performed in the practice?
Are there satellite offices in or out of this area?

TIME COMMITMENTS

What is the usual day in the practice like?
What is the call schedule?
What is the weekend schedule?
How does the practice handle holidays?

REIMBURSEMENT STRUCTURE

What payment mechanisms are used most by this practice?
  Fee for service?
  Capitated systems?
  Medicare?
  Medicaid?
What managed care contracts is this practice involved in?
What are the opportunities for reimbursements for advanced practice nurses with these payors?
What services can I provide that will be reimbursable?

ORGANIZATIONAL STRUCTURE?

Who is the practice manager?
  Have I met with him/her?
Who is the key decision maker in the practice?
  Have I met with him/her?
What is the current organizational structure?
How will an ACNP fit into this structure?

ACNP USAGE

What are the reasons for this practice to consider hiring an ACNP?
What are the contributions that I can make to this practice?
What are the services that I can provide that will improve patient outcomes?
What are the services that I can provide that will increase practice productivity?

PRACTICE STRENGTHS/WEAKNESSES

What is the practice reputation?
  In the community?
  Among other physicians?
  Among nursing staff?

Continued

TABLE 6.3 *Continued*

Is the practice owned by an organization or a hospital?
What is the financial security of the practice?
Does the practice have a 5-year plan?
What is the mission statement of the practice?
Are any mergers or acquisitions pending?
What type of outreach is being accomplished?
What are the plans for growth?

specific questions you need to ask in order to determine the personality of the practice. Compare your personal inventory of knowledge, skills, strengths, and weaknesses with the characteristics of the practice. Now, you have the information to craft the scenario about your vital contributions to the practice.

The outcome of your analysis of personal, marketplace, and practice characteristics is a clear understanding of the power you have to negotiate for what you are worth.

Setting Limits and Goals

Power in a negotiation comes from knowing what you can and cannot accept and deciding ahead of time that you will walk away from the negotiation when the line has been crossed. Setting limits and goals is like developing the endpoints on a continuum of job acceptability. The limits tell you the point at which you will terminate negotiations, and the goals establish the outcomes you want to achieve.

Setting limits requires that you analyze the self-evaluation data within the context of marketplace and practice characteristics and determine what items are nonnegotiable. Remember, you must be prepared to terminate the negotiation if the practice cannot accept a nonnegotiable item. It is a very powerful feeling to know that you are prepared to walk away from the negotiations at a certain predetermined point. Think back in your own experiences, either personal or professional, and you can probably identify a time when you allowed yourself to accept an agreement that was not really acceptable to you. You probably ended up feeling abused and unhappy. These feelings are always the outcome when you sacrifice your principles. Walk away from a negotiation when the terms are unacceptable to you because there *will* be other opportunities. The only limits on options are the ones you create in your own mind.

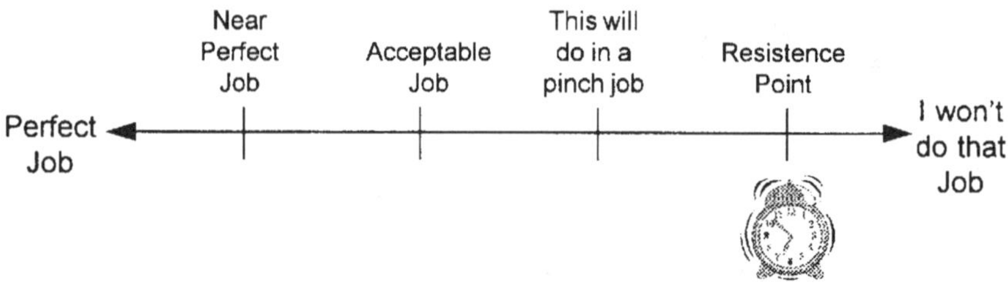

FIGURE 6.1

To help yourself identify other options you have, make a list of potential job opportunities. The bigger it is the more power you possess in a negotiation. Now prioritize this list. What is the next best option if this negotiation fails, and so on? The list becomes an action plan and will help immensely with negotiations because you have identified a very viable alternative plan.

Before entering into negotiations, identify the resistance point or the place very close to your limit (Donaldson & Donaldson, 1996). The resistance point is like a loud bell reminding you that your limit is approaching. Acknowledge the warning, reflect on the negotiations, and determine strategies (see Figure 6.1).

On the other end of the continuum are goals. These are the outcomes that you want to accomplish. When you are negotiating a contract as an ACNP, you are setting up the terms of your next employment relationship. You are also taking a course of action that will influence your professional career. So, goals are both long term and short term. In the short term, you are trying to negotiate a work environment that is both economically and personally satisfying. In the long run, you are negotiating a phase in your professional career that will help you accomplish your ultimate career goals. Both of these needs are important to keep in mind as you set goals. Donaldson and Donaldson (1996) state that useful goals have four characteristics: agreed upon by all involved, specific to the current negotiation, limited in number, and bold but possible to accomplish. Discuss your goals with family, friends, professional colleagues, and mentors because their input will help you clarify your thinking.

Now that you have the ends of the job acceptability continuum established, identify points along the continuum that represent levels of satisfaction with the deal. This exercise will allow you to determine what you can easily give up, what you are willing to give up, what you can be forced to give up, and what you won't give up. With all the preparation completed, it is time to begin negotiations. The next sections describe personal characteristics that are helpful in negotiations.

Managing Emotions

Power in a negotiating situation requires effective cognitive functioning. Strong emotions such as fear, anxiety, anger, frustration, and hurt interfere with cognitive functioning (Herman, 1996). Therefore, managing emotions is an important part of negotiating. The preparation just described has an emotional component to it because being well prepared bolsters confidence. There are a number of other strategies that can be used to prepare emotionally before entering into negotiations. Practice saying positive messages to yourself. Rehearse possible scenarios and decide your response to each. This strategy should keep you from being surprised during negotiations and prepare you to respond thoughtfully.

Managing emotions during negotiations is necessary so that cognitive functioning is at its best. Donaldson and Donaldson (1996) recommend developing a pause button. Developing a pause button requires that you have personal awareness of your emotional state and the impact of this emotional state on cognitive functioning. Then when emotions interfere with cognition, you can press the pause button by asking for a break, pausing and acting pensive, or asking for the negotiations to be rescheduled (Donaldson & Donaldson, 1996). This pause in the action gives you an opportunity to reflect on the events that have just transpired and to determine an appropriate course of action in a less emotional atmosphere.

Listening

Active listening increases power in a negotiation (Donaldson & Donaldson, 1996). It is impossible to negotiate if you do not *hear* what the other person is communicating. By hearing, you have accurate information about the goals, position, and negotiating points of the other person, and knowledge is power. Nurses have a great advantage in this area because the techniques of therapeutic communication such as restating, paraphrasing, reflecting, and asking for more information are just the skills needed in negotiating. If it has been awhile since you practiced these skills, take some time to review the basic principles, practice the techniques, and hone your listening skills.

Communicating Clearly

Clear communication increases power in negotiations. Your communication style can be a valuable asset or a substantial liability when negotiating for an ACNP position. McCallister (1992) identifies two communication styles that are particularly problematic: reflective and candidate. Reflective-style communicators are patient, good listeners, able to tune into others needs, and helpful in solving other's problems. These characteristics probably describe most nurses. Reflective-style communicators tend to withdraw from controversial areas and refrain from communicating what they are really thinking. It is very difficult to have successful negotiations when one party is not communicating clearly.

Candidate-style communicators want to be liked. They communicate in a warm, supportive, and logical manner. They are personable and easy to get along with. They too are not clearly communicating their needs, however. If you possess this style, your need to be liked by the potential employer will overshadow your desire for successfully negotiating aspects of the position, such as an adequate salary. Candidate-style communicators are easy prey for assertive negotiators. Both reflective- and candidate-style communicators should get some help through assertiveness training or mentoring from a person who is a clear communicator. McCallister (1992) recommends that these individuals plan and practice prior to initiation of any negotiations.

When communicating your ideas in written form, you want to ensure that each letter and document is accurately prepared and professionally presented. The content of the written documents is important in expressing the message you intend. In Portfolio Development, below, we describe specific content you want to communicate clearly to a potential employer.

PORTFOLIO DEVELOPMENT

One of the most powerful tools for communicating the value of the ACNP is through the use of a professional portfolio. A portfolio is a formal document that showcases qualifications and expertise, past clinical and professional experiences, and scholarly work. A portfolio contains information to educate potential employers unfamiliar with the scope of ACNP practice. Burgess and Misener (1997) described 10 categories that a portfolio should contain. These categories include: (a) resume, (b) program of study and student experiences (for those entering the job market for the first time), (c) legal regulations, (d) standards and scope of practice for your specialty, (e) samples of scholarly work, (f) sample job description ; (g) reimbursement guidelines; (h) sample list of procedures; (i) hospital privileging information, and (j) sample protocols. In addition, we recommend that an ACNP portfolio include samples of dictations, orders, and other documentation; a listing of professional expenses; and projected income generation.

Developing the portfolio takes time, planning, and work, but once completed it will be a powerful statement of your worth to the organization and will enhance your negotiating position. The following sections provide specific details about the individual categories, elements found in each, and the rationale for inclusion.

Résumé

A concise resume should include educational history, employment history, awards, certifications, professional memberships, specialty expertise, and qualifications relevant to this position. If seeking positions in a variety of practices, you should tailor the resume to highlight the skills most appealing to each potential employer. A resume gives a potential employer a snapshot of your career and qualifications.

Program of Study and Student Experiences

For those entering the job market in advanced practice for the first time, the portfolio should contain information about educational experiences. A complete listing will contain the courses taken along with a brief course description (Burgess & Misener, 1997). Develop a summary of your clinical experiences, such as the total number of contact hours, types of clients managed, age ranges, procedures performed, practice location, and preceptor. Letters of recommendation from past preceptors can also be a strong addition to this category. This discussion is one mechanism to demonstrate the breadth of clinical and theoretical knowledge you have acquired.

Legal Regulations

In this portion of the portfolio, you should include a copy of the nurse practice act and any regulations that pertain to advanced practice nursing in your state. You should describe the process of obtaining advanced practice recognition and prescriptive authority and specify documents that must be provided by the practice. Furnishing this information demonstrates attention to the legal aspects of your practice and provides employers not familiar with advanced practice nursing an opportunity to review the regulations (Hravnak & Magdic, 1997; Burgess & Misener, 1997).

Standards and Scope of Practice for Your Specialty

A complete portfolio should contain the Standards of Clinical Practice and Scope of Practice for the Acute Care Nurse Practitioner (American Nurses Association, 1995). This document outlines the standards of competent care and can serve as the basis for a quality review program and performance appraisal (Burgess & Misener, 1997).

Samples of Scholarly Work

Providing samples of your scholarly work can give the potential employer an idea of your writing skills and potential for other scholarly activities. Submitting publications, abstracts, or papers demonstrates your unique contributions to the practice and sets the stage for negotiating attendance at professional meetings (Burgess & Misener, 1997).

Sample Job Description

This category allows you to develop and present an ideal job description that matches your skills with the practice characteristics (Burgess & Misener, 1997). A job description can assist the employer to put into operation your integration into the practice structure. As you did with the resume, individualize the job description for each practice. The job description should provide information concerning specific responsibilities, daily duties, supervision and collaboration, practice sites, and performance appraisal. Develop a week-long sample schedule as an aid to negotiating time commitments. Be as specific as you can. Levels of responsibility vary, necessitating differing levels of compensation. We recommend developing multiple options. If other ACNPs are currently employed with this practice, their job descriptions may be used as a guideline. Be clear on what you want in this position and do not let existing job descriptions unduly influence your negotiating position.

Sample List of Procedures

State nurse practice acts usually determine the procedures within the scope of ACNP practice (Burgess & Misener, 1997). Your list should include procedures that are commonly performed in your state and local jurisdiction, procedures you have performed under supervision during your educational and work experiences, and procedures you are willing to learn. If you have received special training for specific procedures, provide details regarding that training, the number of procedures completed, the outcomes, and any documentation such as procedure notes or dictations. By presenting this procedure list to a potential employer, you are building a stronger platform for negotiating your scope of practice.

Hospital Privileging Information

Because the ACNP role is so new, many hospitals do not have established procedures for privileging advanced practice nurses. When they encounter a request, hospitals are required to develop a plan for privileging ACNPs. During your preparation, determine the specific approach for each hospital used by the practice. Outline the method for obtaining privileges, the documentation required by the facility, and the fees for application. Being well informed and prepared to answer questions regarding privileging will ameliorate a potential barrier that may impede your negotiations (Hravnak & Magdic, 1997).

Sample Protocols

In many states, advanced practice nurses are required to use protocols or guidelines for practice. Creating a protocol for management of a clinical problem specific to the practice you are considering is a excellent way to demonstrate the scope of practice of an ACNP. If protocol books are available, include a bibliography in your portfolio (Burgess & Misener, 1997). The protocol will demonstrate the clinical responsibilities, diagnostic reasoning, treatment modalities, and patient outcomes that can be expected from ACNP practice.

Samples of Dictations, Orders, and Other Documentation

Present evidence of your advanced practice documentation skills by including samples of dictations, orders, discharge summaries, admission notes, and progress notes specific to the practice population. Remember to maintain patient confidentiality by removing any identifying information. This section of the portfolio can be very powerful in illustrating your clinical expertise.

Professional Expenses

In your portfolio, you should furnish an itemized listing of the professional expenses you expect to have included in your salary and benefits package. The more specific you are in preparing your proposal, the clearer you will communicate your expectations and needs. This document will also serve as a starting point for negotiating your benefits package and thus should be as comprehensive as possible. When listing expenses, take into consideration all one-time and yearly costs associated with your professional practice, maintenance of certifications, licensure, continuing education, liability insurance, and professional organization fees. Some practices may have a standard package but are usually able to adjust it to the needs of the employee. A sample format for expenses is included in Table 6.4.

Projected Income Generation

Determining the benefits of the services you are able to provide and explicitly stating these for your potential employer can be the most difficult part of preparing your portfolio. Much of this portion of the proposal will depend on the system you are entering and the value they place on the various types of services.

Calculation of potential income generation is based on services provided, payment mechanism, and provider mix. It is always advantageous to underestimate your income potential. In a fee for service setting, you will need to determine the levels of service and the charges for each level. If you are expecting to see patients in an office setting estimate the number of patients seen each day times the number of days per week times the number of weeks per year you will be available. Use the lowest reimbursable rate for the level of patient you will regularly manage. A sample calculation can be found in Table 6.5. Inpatient rounds and care can be calculated in the same manner using the average census and reimbursement scheme. Include other contributions such as patient satisfaction, decreased length of stay, reduced yearly hospitalizations, and readmission rates and use these to estimate the impact on patient outcomes and practice operations. If providing services in a capitated

Table 6.4 Professional Expenses

ITEM	**ESTIMATED EXPENSE**
Salary	62,000.00
	re-evaluated in 6 months and annually thereafter. Includes at least 21 days paid vacation and 32 hours paid leave for continuing education. Sick time and additional time off post weekends and call to be discussed.
Liability Insurance	491.00 yearly
	2,000,000/occurrence
	4,000,000 aggregate
Prescriptive Authority	20.00 one-time application fee
DEA #	310.00 one-time application fee
	170.00 yearly
Practice relocation	25.00 one-time fee
License renewal	50.00 yearly
Professional organizations	300.00 yearly
Continuing education	1500.00 yearly
15 contact hours required for certification	
7.5 contact hours required for prescriptive authority	
Journals	200.00 yearly
Beeper	75.00 initial cost, 180.00 yearly
Cellular phone charges	600.00 yearly (50.00/month)
OTHER	
Medical/dental family coverage	8,000.00 yearly
Profit sharing office, staff support, etc.	8,000.00 yearly
TOTAL	**(approximately 39% of base salary)**
One time fees	**480.00**
Ongoing expenses	**89,491.00**

TABLE 6.5 Sample Income Calculation

Determine what you will provide to the physician or potential employer. Just imagine that you would see 3 clients per hour (although you may see 4 or 5).

The charge is $35 per visit. You work only 20 hours per week in the office. (3 patients seen x $35 per visit generated x 20 hours per week equals $2100.)

$2100 per week x 48 weeks equals $100,800 gross income annually. Forty-eight weeks is used in the calculation to adjust for vacation time, and continuing education time.

Now subtract 40% for overhead ($40,320) from your gross income. Overhead calculations may vary. Your annual salary earned just on your office time alone is $60,480.

system, you should identify the specific service you can offer and calculate the impact that service will have on patient outcomes and overall productivity of the practice.

ISSUES IN CONTRACT NEGOTIATION

The goal in any negotiation is for each party to get the most while giving up the least. The only person looking out for your best interest is you! Go into each negotiating situation fully prepared, make sure you discuss all the areas of concern, and have all your questions answered. Shupe (1997) recommends getting a written contract. The contracting process provides a forum to discuss issues of concern. Below are some specific suggestions for terms of the contract. Table 6.6 contains questions that should be asked as you enter contract negotiation.

Contracts are usually for a year, although the length may vary. Your contract should specifically indicate renewal time and renewal terms. Unless you have a renewal date, your contract could automatically roll over to a new year with the same terms. The only way to change the terms of a contract is to ask for a renegotiation or have one scheduled in your contract. Commonly, contracts are renewed 30 days before termination date, and all terms are renewable at that time. The contract needs to specify the review process, including criteria to be used and reviewer (Shupe, 1997).

Many practices and institutions have multiple sites and outreach programs. The contract should indicate the site or sites of employment. If multiple sites are used, you need to determine the costs of travel between sites and who will be responsible for this. Travel time and mile-

TABLE 6.6 Contract Worksheet

CONTRACT TERMS
What is the length of the contract?
How will the terms be renegotiated?
How and when will performance appraisals be conducted?
Who will conduct the performance appraisal?

SITES
Will I be required to practice in multiple sites?
Are these within the state?
What will the travel time and mileage be?
What would the average monthly cost for travel and mileage be?
Will the practice pay for travel time and mileage?
What are the costs of obtaining licensure/recognition in other states?
Will the practice pay for licensure/recognition in the other state(s) ?

SALARY/BENEFITS
Am I paid on a salary or hourly basis?
Will overtime be compensated?
What will the overtime rate be?
Is comp time an alternative to paid overtime?
What are the work week expectations?
What are the call responsibilities?
What Health insurance plan will be provided and at what expense to me?
What dental insurance plan will be provided and at what expense to me?
What life insurance plan is available and at what expense to me?
Will the practice pay for malpractice insurance?
What sick leave policies are in place?
Will I receive pay for sick days?
What are the vacation policies?
Is vacation time paid?
How much advance notice is needed?

CONTINUING EDUCATION & DUES
What amount of continuing education (CE) costs will be reimbursed by the practice?
Who will decide which offering I will attend?
Will I receive travel expenses for CE?
Will I receive paid leave for CE?
How much advance notice is needed?
What amount of professional dues will be reimbursed?
Who will decide the type of professional dues that will be paid?

OUTSIDE EMPLOYMENT
Can I provide any services as outside employment?
Who receives the reimbursement for the services?

TERMINATION
How much notice am I required to give them?
How much notice are they required to give me?

Continued

TABLE 6.6 *Continued*

Who can terminate me?
Is an employer anticompetition clause in the contract?
What is the definition of competition?
What is the restriction on radius?
What is the length of the restriction?
ARBITRATION
Is arbitration required?
Who chooses the arbitrator?
Who pays the arbitrator?
Where is the arbitration conducted?

age should be included in the travel expenses. Your practice sites may also be in different states, necessitating that you be licensed and approved for advanced practice privileges in those states. You need to determine the costs associated with this process and who will be expected to pay the expenses. One option is to have the practice pay for the initial license and applications for advanced practice privileges. Then, you can be responsible for all renewals (Shupe, 1997). Your knowledge of the costs associated with multiple licensures and travel is essential in protecting yourself from assuming a large unexpected expense.

Compensation comes in two forms: salary and benefits. Use the data collected during preparation for the negotiations to determine the relative balance between salary and benefits. Your personal situation will dictate the kinds of benefits you want and need. You should clarify whether you will be paid on a salary or hourly basis and whether overtime hours will be reimbursed differently. Overtime is a reality in health care, especially in acute care. Work week expectations, call responsibilities, and overtime compensation should be stated in the contract (Shupe, 1997).

Remember that negotiating salary in a job interview is quite different from asking for a raise (McCallister, 1992). There are several points that need to be considered as you enter this phase of your contract negotiation. In the job interview, the physician practice is trying to acquire a nurse practitioner to assume responsibility for some of the patient load. At this point in the negotiations, you have the advantage. You are what McCallister (1992) refers to as the "scarce resource" (p. 142). If you were already employed and simply asking for a raise, the practice would already have you, giving the practice the advantage. In addition, employing physicians, hospitals, or managed care organizations may have guidelines or rules governing pay raises for midlevel providers. The last consideration is that federal and state agencies are undergoing maximum cuts in an effort to balance the federal budget, and merit increases are often minimal. Your best opportunity for negotiating salary requirements is at the time you enter the practice.

Health insurance, dental insurance, life insurance, malpractice insurance, sick leave, and vacation time are all areas that require negotiation. Frequently, practices have a standard package or group of programs and policies for these benefits. Make certain you are well informed about the types of benefits, insurance carriers used, amount of coverage, and your part of the expenses. Review any policies related to sick and vacation time, and the reimbursement you will receive when you are on leave.

Continuing education and professional dues are other benefits that should be clarified during negotiation. There are usually yearly caps on the budgeted amount for reimbursement of these expenses. You need to determine who authorizes continuing education, who determines the appropriateness of the offering, and how much advance notice the practice needs in order to provide coverage while you attend a conference. Your reimbursement may depend on approval by your practice partners. You also need to ascertain how your continuing education budget will be affected if the practice asks you to attend a conference. Two options are possible: the expenses can be deducted from your yearly budget or the expenses are covered outside of your yearly cap.

Outside employment issues should be discussed in any negotiation. The practice may require all or a specific portion of any compensation you receive for activities, lectures, or outside employment. You need to understand all limitations on your services outside of your daily responsibilities. One solution is to specify in your contract that when the practice shares in the financial benefits, the practice should share in the malpractice insurance and tax expenses.

Termination terms must be discussed as a part of your contract negotiation. Many contracts have a clause that stipulates that the employer can terminate employment for cause. You as the employee may also be able to resign for cause. You need to determine whether you have this option as part of your contract. Your termination terms should include the amount of notice required by both parties prior to termination and designate the person(s) in the practice with the power to terminate your employment.

Employer anticompetition clauses are frequently found in health care provider contracts. These clauses can significantly restrict your ability to practice after you leave the organization. You could be blocked from practicing or competing within a specific mile radius of your former employer for a specific period of time. Review this clause carefully to determine all of the restrictions that may be imposed. Your goal in the negotiation is to get this clause as narrow as possible in terms of time and distance, if not deleted altogether. Within the wording of the clause, "competition" should be clearly defined. The clause should not be worded in a way that would restrict your ability to get a job.

Arbitration and mediation terms are frequently found in contractual agreements. You need to determine your ability to sue your employer for breech of contract. Many contracts require that employee and employer go to arbitration and restrict legal action in the event of a dispute. In this case, you need to identify the person(s) responsible for choosing the arbitrator, the person paying for the arbitrator, and the location of the arbitration. Your attention to this issue will prevent any arbitration from being arranged without your input, at significant cost to you, and in a location that puts you at a disadvantage.

Negotiating a contract will require in-depth discussion of all the terms and careful review of the actual document. Whether or not you need to consult a lawyer depends on how much support you need, your experience with employment contracts, and the complexity of the contract.

DEALING WITH RESISTANCE TO THE ROLE

Change generates resistance and because the ACNP role is new, there will be resistance to the role. Possible sources of resistance include staff nurses, advanced practice nurses, hospital administrators, physician assistants, physicians, and consumers. Overcoming the resistance requires that you discover the specific reasons for resistance in each group and plan appropriate strategies. In the following, we discuss some of the general strategies that ACNPs can use to increase their power and decrease resistance to the role.

A major problem for ACNPs is a lack of understanding about the roles that advanced practice nurses play (O'Malley, Cummings, & King, 1996). There is confusion about knowledge and skills, scope of practice, and differentiation of abilities from similar providers. This confusion may lead to negative attitudes. Promulgation of information about the role is the strategy of choice. Develop a fact sheet to use when communicating with any potential employer or consumer of ACNP services. The fact sheet should contain clear and concise talking points that highlight the ACNP's contributions to patient care, differentiate the ACNP from competing providers, and clarify misinformation common in the community. Networking with the state nurses association and the advanced practice council is helpful. If the fact sheet were to be used by many of the nurses in the state, dissemination of accurate and consistent information would be greatly enhanced. Although information about the role is helpful, findings from research that document the outcomes of ACNP practice are much more powerful (Buppert, 1995). There are a number of studies that have demonstrated the quality outcomes that are typical of nurse practitioner care. Unfortunately, most of these studies include primary care nurse practitioners. There are some preliminary studies that demonstrate positive outcomes for ACNPs, however. Write abstracts for each study and use these, along with the fact sheet, when you discuss ACNP practice with potential employers. It is essential that ACNPs conduct and report findings from studies that measure the impact of ACNP care on patient outcomes (Hadley, 1996; Hravnak, Rosenzweig, & Baldisseri, 1996). There is no better way to overcome resistance to the role than to demonstrate competence and expertise. When you possess knowledge and skills that contribute substantially to improved patient outcome, the arguments put forward by the restraining forces have less credibility. Use the preparation process and the professional portfolio to detail your strengths. If you identify a weakness in your knowledge and skills that will impact negatively on your negotiating position, institute a plan to remedy the deficiency. Continue to gain expertise by attending conferences, taking courses, and using informal learning opportunities (Hadley, 1996). The goal is to possess so much expertise that the system cannot get along without you.

Legal and regulatory barriers to advanced practice are common and border on restraint of trade. ACNPs need to get politically active. Work with the state board to eliminate barriers to advanced practice and network with other ACNPs (O'Malley, Cummings, & King, 1996).

Attitude and presence are powerful assets that you have to counteract resistance to the ACNP role. Remember that you were prepared for a discipline, not a job (O'Malley, Cummings, & King, 1996). This socialization should have happened while you were in school. Members of a discipline are confident, competent, and professional. They dress and act as if they have power, and they use power effectively. They expect responsibility, respect, and collaboration. When you dress, act, and communicate as a professional, others pay attention!

SUMMARY

One of the outcomes of health care reform is the recognition that midlevel providers are needed to care for acutely ill patients. Nursing responded to this need by developing the ACNP. ACNPs are negotiating for positions in an unstable health-care system: the role is new and evolving, opportunities are great, and competition is stiff. Negotiating skills are essential. The worksheets and professional portfolio development structure your preparation for negotiation. The strategies for listening, communicating, obtaining an advantageous contract, and overcoming resistance to the role provide a framework for actions you can take to negotiate for what you are worth. With these tools, you can create a powerful negotiating position.

REFERENCES

American Nurses Association & American Association of Critical Care Nurses. (1995). *Standards of clinical practice and scope of practice for the acute care nurse practitioner.* Washington, DC: American Nurses Publishing.

Buppert, C.K. (1995). Justifying nurse practitioner existence: Hard facts to hard figures. *Nurse Practitioner, 20,* 43–48.

Burgess, S., & Misener, T. R. (1997). *Clinical Excellence for Nurse Practitioners, 1,* 468–471.

Clochesy, J.M., Daly, B.J., Idemoto, B.K., Steel, J., & Fitzpatrick, J.J. (1994). Preparing advanced practice nurses for acute care. *American Journal of Critical Care, 3,* 255–259.

Donaldson, M.C., & Donaldson, M. (1996). *Negotiating for dummies.* Foster City, CA: IDG Books Worldwide, Inc.

Hadley, E.H. (1996). Nursing in the political and economic marketplace: Challenges for the 21st century. *Nursing Outlook, 44,* 6–10.

Herman, J.A. (1996, March). *Testing of the visual analogue scale to measure anxiety in critically ill patients.* Paper presented at the Tenth Annual Southern Nursing Research Society Conference, Miami Beach, FL.

Hravnak, M., & Magdic, K. (1997). Marketing the acute care nurse practitioner. *Clinical Excellence for Nurse Practitioners, 1,* 9–13.

Hravnak, M., Rosenzweig, M.Q., & Baldisseri, M. (1996). Current questions with regard to acute care nurse practitioner preparation and role implementation. *AACN Clinical Issues, 7,* 289–299.

Hupcey, J.E. (1993). Factors and work settings that may influence nurse practitioner practice, *Nursing Outlook, 41,* 181–185.

McCallister, L. (1992). *I wish I'd said that: How to talk your way out of trouble and into success.* New York: John Wiley & Sons, Inc.

O'Malley, J., Cummings, S., & King, C.S. (1996). The politics of advanced practice. *Nursing Administration Quarterly, 20,* 62–72

Shupe, D. (1997, April). *Negotiating an individual contract.* Paper presented at the Fifth Annual Acute Care Nurse Practitioner Consensus Conference, Myrtle Beach, SC.

Wilken, M. (1995). State regulatory board structure, regulations, and nurse practitioner availability. *Nurse Practitioner, 20,* 68–74.

7

Formulating the Acute Care Nurse Practitioner Job Description

Lynn A. Kelso

ESTABLISHING THE ROLE

Initiating a practice as an acute care nurse practitioner (ACNP) can be a challenging task. Because the ACNP role is new, employing agencies are often unfamiliar with the role components of the ACNP. As a result, ACNPs are often involved in outlining their job description. The purpose of this chapter is to discuss aspects of ACNP role development and formulation of the ACNP job description.

The majority of graduating ACNPs will need to establish the ACNP role within an acute care setting. Occasionally, a nurse may enter an ACNP program in light of a new advanced practice position in the respective institution. Because the ACNP role is a relatively new advanced practice role, however, most ACNP positions will need to be formulated.

Educating both practice setting administrators and physicians is of utmost importance in establishing a role. For most ACNPs the education process begins while they are enrolled in their graduate program and completing their clinical practicums. By becoming a member of the clinical team as a student, you can educate the team in that setting about the advantages of employing the ACNP; this could be a powerful asset in establishing a future ACNP role in that practice setting. Convincing the members of the medical team that you can be an asset is of greatest importance because they are who you will be working with most closely in a collaborative role.

Educating the practice setting administration is also imperative if the role is to be developed in a way that uses the ACNP's skills optimally. Although physicians are becoming more aware of economic issues related to health care, administrators have always been interested in health-care costs. Although there is little research presently available showing the benefits of employing an ACNP, data exists that show the benefits of employing nurse practitioners in a primary care setting. Using these data and generalizing them to the acute care setting may help to illustrate the benefits of employing ACNPs within acute care settings.

FINDING EMPLOYMENT

Presently, ACNP positions are not widely advertised in local newspapers. Professional publications usually are the best source for ACNP position advertisements. These positions, along with those that may be advertised on the Internet, however, may require a change of location. If relocating is not an option, review the want ads in the local newspaper. Review the nurse practitioner openings as well as those for physician assistants (PAs). Although many physicians are not familiar with ACNPs, they are familiar with PAs. Identify any PA position that may be of interest to you as a prospective job and inquire about it. You should speak with whoever will be supervising the position and be prepared to compare and contrast the roles of the ACNP and PA. Identify what advantages there would be to hiring an ACNP for the position and what your vision of the ACNP role is. The key is in identifying what needs the role will fulfill. For example, if a cardiothoracic surgery service is interested in hiring someone who can specifically work in the operating room with them, you may not be particularly interested. If you can give them a clear picture of what role you can play, however, they may be willing to modify their job expectations.

Obtaining employment soon after graduation is essential. This will allow the ACNP to function in the role and gain experience. Waiting for the perfect position may not be an option; delaying employment may affect future job opportunities.

FORMULATING THE ROLE

Assessing an employer's perceptions of the ACNP role is paramount to evaluating a potential position. Some employers are eager to hire an ACNP because they believe that the ACNP can serve as a replacement for downsizing the medical resident staff. Although the ACNP role is focused on direct management of patient care, ACNPs are not physician replacements. Rather, they bring a cohesive element to care, providing comprehensive care management, overseeing patient and family teaching, and consulting with other members of the health-care team to ensure that all aspects of patient care are accomplished efficiently. Additionally, the ACNP may have job responsibilities in staff education, quality monitoring projects, and research. Communication about the various components of the ACNP role becomes important in ensuring that the role you are hired for will allow for full use of ACNP capabilities.

An essential document for all ACNPs is the "Standards of Clinical Practice and Scope of Practice for the Acute Care Nurse Practitioner" (American Nurses Association, 1995). The scope of practice, role in acute care, and standards of clinical practice for the ACNP are outlined in the document. It can prove to be a valuable resource for translating role components and for developing the ACNP job description.

DEVELOPING THE ACUTE CARE NURSE PRACTITIONER JOB DESCRIPTION

Whether an employing institution has an ACNP job description which needs refining or they will expect your involvement in developing one, active participation in outlining role responsibilities and components is a distinct advantage of the newness of the ACNP position. The general job description should be broad and include a description of the ACNP role, the qualifications required, and the responsibilities and functions of the role. It should also include a statement about supervision and guidance of the role. An example of a job description for the ACNP can be found in Table 7.1.

A general description of the ACNP role may simply state the nature and purpose of the work involved in a very broad definition, providing

TABLE 7.1 ACNP Job Description

Title: Acute Care Nurse Practitioner (ACNP)
Department: Nursing

QUALIFICATIONS

1. Licensure as a professional nurse in the Commonwealth of Kentucky
2. Certification as an advanced registered nurse practitioner (ARNP) in the Commonwealth of Kentucky
   a. certification as an ACNP by the ANA certification exam
   b. certification as an adult nurse practitioner (ANP) or family nurse practitioner (FNP) by the ANA certification exam with a minimum of 500 hr clinical practice in an acute care setting within the previous 2 years
3. Graduation from an accredited ACNP program or from an accredited ANP/FNP program and eligible to sit for the ACNP certification exam by American Nurses Association.
4. Minimum 3 years nursing experience with 2 years experience in area of practice
5. Masters degree in nursing
6. ACLS preferred, required within 12 months of employment

NATURE AND PURPOSE OF WORK

The ACNP is to provide advanced nursing care across the continuum of acute care services to patients who are acutely or critically ill. The ACNP functions as a member of the medical care management team. The focus of the ACNP is to provide restorative care by

1. providing holistic, comprehensive patient care across an identified continuum
2. providing consistency within the medical care management team
3. consolidating and coordinating optimal resources, with the multidisciplinary team, for acceptable patient/family outcomes

The short-term goal is the stabilization of the patient, minimizing complications and providing physical and psychological care measures. The long-term goal is to restore the patient/family to maximal health potential and evaluate risk factors in achieving this outcome or providing for a peaceful, dignified death.

Medical diagnostic, therapeutic, and management functions are instituted under medical supervision using protocols developed by each service. Clinical privileges for each ACNP are recommended by the supervising physician to the Medical Credentialing Committee.

The ACNP's ability to engage in activities that normally constitute the practice of nursing is not hindered by the credentialing process, provided the ACNP has the preparation, knowledge, and experience necessary to execute the practice.

The ACNP may be unit based, service/specialty based, or hospital based.

Responsibilities and Functions

There are five areas of advanced practice within which the ACNP may function: (1) direct, comprehensive patient care, (2) systems management, (3) education, (4) research, and (5) publication and professional leadership.

Direct, comprehensive patient care. The ACNP diagnoses medical conditions, plans and implements interventions, evaluates patient response while continually altering the plan of care. This is accomplished under direction of and in collaboration with a physician supervisor or designated attending physician.

Continued

TABLE 7.1 *Continued*

1. Assembles complete medical data base, including health history and physical examination, upon admission of selected patients
2. Assesses selected patients using physically and technologically derived data, including the evaluation of diagnostic test results
3. Under the direction of and in consultation/collaboration with the supervising physician, or designee, diagnoses medical conditions and plans and orders medical consultations, therapies, and interventions based upon assessment and protocol. These include, but are not limited to, medications; diagnostic tests; respiratory care, including ventilator management; nutrition; fluid and electrolyte support; blood/blood products.
4. Performs invasive diagnostic and therapeutic procedures based on the needs of the specific patient population and as determined collaboratively by the ACNP, the supervising physician, and the service or unit director and approved by the medical credentialing committee
5. Evaluates and analyzes the patient's response to disease processes and therapeutic interventions and alters the plan of care as needed
6. Documents all assessment data, orders, interventions, results, and evaluations within the patient's medical record; begins and documents discharge planning in a timely fashion
7. Participates in medical team rounds and presents selected patients
8. Facilitates the development of protocols for service/unit that will guide the practice of the ACNP
9. Provides information, education, and support to patients and families; facilitates communication between patients, family members, and members of the multidisciplinary team. Includes both patients and family members in planning care and discharge
10. Provides continuity of care within the service/unit
11. Serves as a consultant and resource person to members of the multidisciplinary team, to facilitate/coordinate patient care delivery, based on expertise in area of specialty
12. Serves as patient/family advocate and facilitates ethical decision making within patient care
13. Facilitates efficient movement of the patient within the health-care system to ensure quality and cost-effective care

Systems Management

1. Promotes and practices economical and effective health care
2. Participates in strategic planning for the service, department, or hospital, including recruitment and retention activities of the medical center
3. Serves on University of Kentucky committees related to ACNP/ARNP utilization, including regularly updating medical management protocols
4. Exhibits behaviors that reflect commitment to the philosophy and vision of the University, the medical center, and the departments of nursing and medicine
5. Participates in the assessment, development, implementation, and evaluation of quality improvement programs, standards of practice, policies and procedures

TABLE 7.1 *Continued*

Research

1. Participates in medical and nursing research projects, including the presentation and publication of findings
2. Integrates research findings into practice
3. Conducts clinical investigations based on practice or quality improvement issues
4. Assists in locating potential funding sources to support investigation of clinical issues or program development

Education

1. Participates in activities that contribute to the education of health-care professionals, including presenting and publishing
2. Provides appropriate patient and family education
3. Serves as a mentor and preceptor to nursing students, medical students, and new orientees and provides on-going feedback
4. Identifies the need for and conducts educational programs for the hospital staff
5. Establishes goals for own professional growth
6. Attends continuing education programs
7. Maintains credentialing and required certification and documents evidence of continued competency in the areas of medical diagnoses, therapeutics, invasive procedures, and management

Publication and Professional Leadership

1. Participates in professional organizations
2. Serves on departmental and interdisciplinary committees
3. Engages in community service
4. Disseminates nursing knowledge through presentation and publication
5. Completes self-evaluation annually

Supervision and Guidance

The Acute Care Nurse Practitioner is accountable to and evaluated by the Associate Director of Nursing. Input is also sought from the supervising physician and designees and nursing and other members of the health-care team.

Note. From Ackerman, M.H., Norsen, L., Martin, B., Wiedrich, J., Kitzman, H.J. (1996). Development of a model of advanced practice. *American Journal of Critical Care, 5*(1), 68–73. Adapted with permission.

comprehensive, holistic care to a select population of patients within a selected area of the institution.

Qualifications should include educational level, state and national certifications required, and experience expected prior to applying for the job. The education should be at the master's level. If there is a great deal of research involved in the position, there may be a need for a doctorally prepared ACNP. There may also be a requirement to have successfully completed the national ACNP certification exam. Although passing a national certification exam may not be required within the state for certification as a nurse practitioner, it may be required, or preferred, for the position. Other certifications may include advanced cardiac life support (ACLS) or advanced trauma life support (ATLS) prior to employment or within a particular time frame after taking the position. There may be a requirement for previous ACNP experience or a minimum number of years of experience in nursing.

Functions and responsibilities of the role can be individualized for your particular role. For example, it may be important to identify the percentage of time that will be spent on direct patient care, research, education, and publishing.

Included in this portion of the job description may be a section highlighting the amount of supervision that is required for particular procedures. The job description should delineate which procedures the ACNP can complete independently and which procedures require direct physician supervision. There may be differing levels of supervision for specific procedures. For example, there may be no need for a physician to be on site for patient assessment, whereas for invasive procedures, such as the placement of a central venous line or intubation of a patient, the physician's presence may be required. As the ACNP gains experience, these levels of supervision may change, but there may be some procedures that will always require direct supervision by the physician. If these levels of supervision are not discussed within the job description, they will need to be addressed within the credentialing procedure of the hospital. There should be a collaborative effort between you and the physician in determining the levels of supervision for particular procedures.

When determining the levels of supervision for invasive procedures, such as arterial line placement or endotracheal intubation, there should be some initial evaluation process. This may be as simple as having the supervising physician complete a procedure evaluation form. This form should state that you performed the procedure with proper technique including assessment of complications and corresponding appropriate actions initiated (Table 7.2). The procedure evaluation forms may serve as important future documentation. Many institutions require a particular number of procedures to be done under supervision before they can be done independently. For example, 25 central line placements may be required before direct supervision is not required.

There may also be a contingency written into either the job description or the credentialing process that states the physicians with whom

TABLE 7.2 Example Procedure Evaluation Form

Name: ______________________	Date:			
Supervisor signature:				
ASEPSIS	yes	no	N/A	comments
1. washed hands				
2. site prepared appropriately				
3. sterile technique throughout procedure				
ARTERIAL CATH PLACEMENT				
1. appropriate indication/site				
2. site used				
3. appropriate landmarks, assessed collateral blood flow (radial)				
4. correct equipment used				
5. correct technique (including suturing)				
6. number of attempts				
VENOUS ACCESS				
1. appropriate indication/site				
2. site used				
3. catheter used				
4. appropriate landmarks				
5. correct equipment used				
6. correct technique (including suturing)				
7. X-ray ordered (if appropriate)				
8. number of attempts				

Additional rows can be added to address other procedures that are being done by the ACNP. These might include pulmonary artery catheter flotation, chest tube insertion, and intubation. The evaluation form can then be altered as appropriate for the practice.

you will be collaborating or by whom you will be supervised. This is important, especially on services that have multiple attending physicians who rotate on the service.

Other role components, such as education, quality monitoring, research, systems management, and professional leadership, should be outlined in the job description.

The availability of time and money for professional meetings and conferences should also be delineated in the job description. Although some states do not require continuing education, other states and national certification renewal do. ACNPs should negotiate for work time and possibly monetary compensation for continuing education. This will facilitate certification renewal and benefit the institution by keeping you well informed on current practices. Chapter 6 by Herman, Selph, Knox,

Nussbaum, and Franklin in this book discusses specific issues related to negotiating aspects of the ACNP job.

The institution's policy and procedure guidelines should also outline the ACNP practice capabilities. Establishing practice protocols is also recommended. Within an institution, protocols may exist for "midlevel providers" such as PAs that may be modified to include the ACNP. Developing protocols specific to ACNP practice is desired and is often required by accreditation agencies and state nurse practice acts.

SUMMARY

As with any new role, establishing yourself as an ACNP will be a challenging but rewarding experience. Formulating a comprehensive job description can ensure that the role uses fully the ACNP capabilities. If a job description exists, careful scrutiny and requests for revisions may be indicated prior to securing a new position that meets your expectations. It will take patience and perseverance in order to begin your new role as an ACNP, but you will be creating a role that holds much promise for a fulfilling career in this new area of advanced practice nursing.

REFERENCES

American Nurses Association. (1995). *Standards of Clinical Practice and Scope of Practice for the Acute Care Nurse Practitioner.* Washington, DC: ANA/AACN.

8

Evaluation of the Acute Care Nurse Practitioner's Role

Helen Stupak Shah and Dori Taylor Sullivan

The purpose of this chapter is to describe a framework for the evaluation of the acute care nurse practitioner (ACNP) role and to review evaluation findings currently available. As with any new health care provider role, the ACNP will profoundly affect the care patients receive, the roles of other health care providers, and the system of health-care delivery. A systematic and comprehensive assessment of the ACNP role and practice will contribute to the optimal performance of an evolving role that promises to play a key role in the redesign of health care.

This chapter provides a brief historical review of the development and the implementation of the ACNP role and its implication for their evaluation, followed by an overview of evaluation methods and frameworks. Finally, evaluation works to date are summarized, and specific recommendations regarding further evaluation of ACNPs are provided.

BACKGROUND

The Nurse Practitioner movement started in the 1960s with Ford and Silver's introduction of pediatric nurse practitioners in Colorado (Mallison, 1993; Silver & McAtee, 1988; Silver, Ford, & Day, 1968). This new role expanded in time to encompass midwifery and family, adult, and other nursing specialties but remained largely a role practiced external to acute care institutions, focused on ambulatory care, and concentrated among medically under-served populations. The lone exception to this pattern was the neonatal nurse practitioner, who quickly became indispensable in the care of neonates in the neonatal intensive care units. The changes within the health-care industry in the twilight of the 20th century precipitated the need for a similar type of practitioner within hospitals. The ACNP became a reality within hospital settings.

Role differences do exist among different ACNPs geographically, across the country, locally among hospitals, and individually among practitioners. There are strong commonalities among the ACNP role, however. ACNPs are proficient in advanced physical assessment, diagnostic reasoning, ordering and interpreting various diagnostic tests and procedures, prescribing medications, and executing therapeutic interventions. Typically, ACNPs carry a patient caseload of anywhere between 2 and 10 patients. They admit patients to their respective services through referral and initiate and manage the hospitalization phase for a variety of patients. In some instances, ACNPs can admit patients directly through affiliation with physician associates holding admitting privileges at their hospitals of choice. In these instances, as well as when hospital based, ACNPs are subject to the process of credentialing and privileging through the medical and nursing departments of their respective institutions.

Implications for Acute Care Nurse Practitioner Evaluation

Any approach to evaluation of ACNPs must be multifaceted and take into consideration a variety of interests and perspectives on the situation. Some work has been completed on ACNP evaluation and an overview of this material is reported elsewhere in this book (see chapter 2). Ingersoll (1995) describes a major problem in ACNP evaluation: disappearance of the role boundary between practitioner and physician practice as the integration of care is perfected. In other words, when care improves in efficiency and quality, role distinctions are more difficult to discern. Thus, evaluation is limited to patient results rather than to individual role contribution. In addition, it is difficult for evaluators to identify the normative or comparison group in which to compare ACNPs.

EVALUATION OVERVIEW

Evaluation may be generally defined as a systematic assessment of the value, worth, and effectiveness of a designated program, role, or intervention. The field of program evaluation is described more specifically as a diligent investigation, using behavioral science research principles and methods, of an entity's characteristics and merits (Fink, 1993; Rossi & Freeman, 1993).

The emergence of the ACNP role may be considered as a "program" or "intervention" for the purpose of evaluating the outcomes and impact of this change. The introduction of a new role into the health-care team is expected to affect not only patients but also the other members of the team and the system within which care is provided. In evaluating the ACNP role, it is critical to identify and explain the specific evaluation goals and the aspects of the role or program that will be addressed. For the purposes of this chapter, one may assume that program and role evaluation are synonymous.

In evaluation terms, "characteristics" refers to descriptive information that provides the context for analyzing and interpreting other evaluation data. "Program merits" (Fink, 1993) refers to the worthiness of goals, achievement of standards of effectiveness, and benefits to participants or stakeholders, or both. An evaluation of program objectives and the extent to which they have been achieved along with review and documentation of program activities (including implementation and management) provides yet another dimension.

Finally, program outcomes and impact are critical evaluation parameters. Outcomes evaluation is the actual change or progress that was accomplished as a result of the program under evaluation. Impact evaluation considers the scope of the program effects, duration of its outcomes, and the extent of influence on other settings or situations. Table 8.1 shows specific examples of these terms for the evaluation of the ACNP. A program evaluation typically consists of the following: defining the program and identifying stakeholders; developing relevant, priority questions about the program; setting standards of effectiveness (measurable criteria to define effectiveness); designing the evaluation and selecting participants; collecting data; analyzing and interpreting the data; and reporting the results.

In most, if not all, evaluations, it is useful to consider a stakeholder analysis. A stakeholder is anyone who has an investment in or will be affected by the program. Every program has multiple stakeholder groups

TABLE 8.1 Evaluation Terms

Characteristics	Gender, age, marital status, nursing specialty, education level
Merits	Delivery of high-quality, cost-effective health care with easy access
Objectives & Activities	
Focus on ACNP education	Curriculum, amount of clinical hours
Focus on ACNP skills	Performance of core competencies
Outcomes	Patient health status and satisfaction
Impact	Relationships with other health providers; use of ACNPs in various settings and specialties
Expenses & Costs	Comparative costs for education, salaries, care delivery, etc.

that either directly participate or become interested in the evaluation process and its results (Rossi & Freeman, 1993). Representative stakeholder groups include policy and decision makers, program sponsors, evaluation sponsor(s), target participants and recipients of services, program management, program staff, evaluators, program competitors, and contextual stakeholders. Relevant stakeholders related to the ACNP role include patients (service recipients), payors (decision makers and contextual stakeholders), physicians (program competitors and program sponsors), health-care and nurse administrators (program management), staff nurses (program staff), and other advanced practice nurses (may be program sponsors, managers, staff, or competitors). Additionally, one might also consider the health-care system and other members of the health-care team as stakeholders.

Stakeholders tend to differ in their perspective of a program under evaluation. In designing evaluations, the evaluator must consider the relative standing and importance of each principal stakeholder group to ensure that the evaluation provides answers to the most compelling evaluation questions. A stakeholder assessment also sensitizes the evaluator to opinions and likely reactions to evaluation results.

Setting standards of effectiveness involves establishing measurable criteria that relate to the program merits claimed. The standards established must be appropriate to the program, measurable with reasonable validity and reliability, and credible. After standards are established, an evaluation design that includes specific plans for selecting participants and collecting data is created.

After the data have been collected and analyzed, the results are reported. Evaluation results are typically written into a formal written report and conveyed through a variety of oral presentations to various stakeholder groups.

Structure-Process-Outcome Evaluation Framework

Another approach to organizing evaluation and quality assessment with which health providers may be more familiar uses the three categories of structure, process, and outcomes (Johnson & Olesinski, 1995). Assessment of the *structure* of inputs to a program is somewhat analogous to program characteristics. *Process* evaluation refers to how a program or role is implemented or performed and includes all activities surrounding the program. Finally, *outcomes* evaluation is concerned with the results of the program or role as they relate to the goals and objectives and to the needs of policy and decision makers. Related terms are formative versus summative evaluation, with formative evaluation involving one or more assessment during the *process* of implementation and summative evaluation looking at the *outcomes* or results.

Examples of specific evaluation variables in these categories related to advanced practice nurses have been described in a meta-analysis of nurse practitioners and nurse midwives (Brown & Grimes, 1993). The *process* indicators for rates of drug prescription and number of laboratory test ordered were included for comparison with physician practice. In the *outcomes* domain, resolution of patient pathological conditions and functional status were measured and compared. Financial comparisons included *outcome* measures, such as hospital length of stay (which is directly correlated with costs), and *process* measures, such as the number of provider visits in the ambulatory setting (in a fee-for-service environment).

A systematic approach to the evaluation of aspects of the ACNP role and practice will ensure that the following evaluation expectations are met:

1. Provide timely, relevant, and accurate information as a basis for decision making related to ACNP effectiveness and efficiency
2. Consider the desired outcomes from the perspective of principal stakeholder groups
3. Assess all major aspects of the program or role
4. Use a variety of methods and sources of data to enhance reliability and validity (including patient records and clinical resource consumption, interviews, observations, etc.)
5. Include appropriate data sampling that reflects the time frames of interest, for example, baseline data, implementation changes, and resulting outcomes of the ACNP role and practice
6. Be cost effective, efficient, and credible

SPECIFIC ACUTE CARE NURSE PRACTITIONER EVALUATIONS

The published body of knowledge encompasses self-efficacy in relation to specific competencies and elements of practitioner work (Shah, Bruttomesso, Taylor Sullivan, & Lattanzio, 1997), self-report on role activities and competencies (Kleinpell, 1997), and recommendations for ongoing and long-range evaluation (Ingersoll, 1995).

Self-Efficacy

The concept of self-efficacy refers to the perception one has of one's own degree of mastery of some area under evaluation or how well one functions in a given situation (Bandura, 1977). To function well, both skills and belief in them must be present. Therefore, self-efficacy tools or questionnaires have been developed and used in role evaluation. The use of self-efficacy tools in role evaluation is useful because they involve not only knowing what to do in a situation but also the integration of cognitive, social, and behavioral subskills for a course of action. Self-efficacy questionnaires may be constructed in such a way as to capture self-performance in terms of specific skills or procedures. Self-efficacy, however, is concerned more with the judgments one has about the skills than the skills themselves. Correlations between self-efficacy and behavioral outcomes have been proposed and documented (Froman & Owen, 1991; Bernal & Froman, 1987). As such, self-efficacy serves as a useful concept in evaluating the role of the ACNP. A self-report, self-efficacy–based instrument was developed collaboratively at the University of Connecticut School of Nursing and Health Center. A copy of the instrument is shown in Table 8.2.

Using this instrument, Shah et al. (1997) reported findings indicating an increase in self-efficacy related to increased clinical experience. This was evident even in areas that are already familiar to staff nurses and, therefore, assumed to already be at a high level of self-efficacy, such as interpreting laboratory or nutritional values and hemodynamic settings.

Performance Evaluation

The evaluation of performance (performance review) is central to all institutional employment situations. For professionals it permits an opportunity to examine goals, review achievements, accept criticism, and

TABLE 8.2 Self-Efficacy Questionnaire Used to Evaluate ACNPs

1. Are you currently responsible for management of the care of patients in collaboration with your preceptor or designated physician? Yes ____ No ____
2. If you answered yes above, how many patients are you managing? (specify)___

PLEASE RATE YOUR RESPONSES TO THE FOLLOWING ITEMS WITH THIS SCALE:

1	**2**	**3**	**4**	**5**	**6**	**7**
Not at all confident		Confident in some situations			Very confident	

3. Where do you feel you are *now* in terms of your preparation to practice as an ACNP?	1 2 3 4 5 6 7
4. Where do you feel you were *6 months ago* in terms of your preparation for the ACNP role?	1 2 3 4 5 6 7
5. How confident will you be *in 6 months* to practice as an ACNP?	1 2 3 4 5 6 7
6. How confident are you in taking a health history?	1 2 3 4 5 6 7
7. How confident are you in performing a physical examination?	1 2 3 4 5 6 7
8. How confident are you in documenting your findings?	1 2 3 4 5 6 7
9. How skilled are you in arriving at a medical diagnosis?	1 2 3 4 5 6 7
10. How confident are you in determining appropriate nursing diagnoses to be discussed and referred to the primary nurse?	1 2 3 4 5 6 7
11. How knowledgeable are you in choosing appropriate diagnostic tests?	1 2 3 4 5 6 7
12. How comfortable are you in interpreting their results?	1 2 3 4 5 6 7
13. How competent are you in formulating a therapeutic plan?	1 2 3 4 5 6 7
14. How competent are you in writing orders in response to a problem?	1 2 3 4 5 6 7

15. Are any body systems causing you particular concern when taking a health history?

General	___	Skin	___
Head	___	Eyes	___
Ears	___	Nose/sinuses	___
Mouth/throat/neck	___	Breasts	___
Lungs	___	Heart	___
GI tract	___	Urinary tract	___
Peripheral vascular	___	Musculoskeletal	___
Nervous	___	Endocrine	___
Hematology	___	Mental status	___
Reproductive			
Male ___		Female ___	

16. Are any body systems causing you particular concern when doing a physical exam?

General	___	Skin	___

Continued

TABLE 8.2 *Continued*

Head	___	Eyes	___
Ears	___	Nose/sinuses	___
Mouth/throat/neck	___	Breasts	___
Lungs	___	Heart	___
GI tract	___	Urinary tract	___
Peripheral vascular	___	Musculoskeletal	___
Nervous	___	Endocrine	___
Hematologic	___	Mental status	___
Genitoreproductive			
Male	___	Female	___

17. Are any other areas of assessment causing you any particular concern?

Laboratory values	___	Imaging results	___
Pathology results	___	Surgical reports	___
Nutritional values	___	Drug sensitivity	___
Hemodynamic values	___	Ventilatory settings	___
Other (specify)			

18. Please tell us anything else you feel we should know in order to evaluate this program.

Note. From the University of Connecticut School of Nursing and Health Center, Storrs, CT. Adapted with permission.

renegotiate priorities with supervisors. For those individuals who are employed in physician multispecialty or group practice situations, performance evaluation tends to be less formalized and possibly sporadic or absent, resulting in lack of written criteria with which to judge progress.

When considering performance evaluation one should also take into account data available from other individuals with whom the ACNP has contact. This is particularly important when the ACNP has reporting pathways to other professionals, for example, physicians. Physicians are accustomed to evaluating the performance of house staff assigned to their services for the purposes of learning proficiency. House staff require evaluation as *students* of medicine. ACNPs require evaluation as *practitioners* of nursing: their ability to coordinate care, collaborate with other care providers, and expedite positive patient outcomes. Often the collaboration piece is overlooked in the intensity of examination of patient-driven outcomes.

The basis of most performance evaluation lies within the performance (job) description. It includes a summary of the purpose for the position, the reporting structure, and expected behaviors. Ideally, the methods of evaluation are also stipulated and usually contain elements of self-reporting and input from supervisors and colleagues. An example of the ACNP performance description in use at the University of Connecticut Health Center is provided in Table 8.3.

In 1995, the University of Connecticut Health Center conducted a review with an additional component that permitted input from other role players interacting with ACNPs. Staff nurses, clinical nurse specialists, unit managers, and physicians were asked to provide data. Survey forms were adapted to each specific group with Likert style and open-ended questions. A copy of the survey, showing items specific to the different nurse groups used, is provided in Table 8.4.

Shah et al. (1997) reported very good to excellent performance from the ACNPs in their study group. Item analysis indicated that areas in need of strengthening were related to the educative, consultative, and professional development role factors. As with self-efficacy, increases in focal areas of performance occur over time and *after* mastery of the clinical behaviors has been achieved. The ACNP participants in the study group recognized a need to increase their consultative and research activities, but they gave priority to areas of patient care management. Evaluators are cautioned to examine the length of service or time since initial ACNP preparation and to factor these data into their results.

Competencies

An important aspect of ACNP evaluation may include an evaluation of specific competencies. As more programs are developed, similarities appear in the expectations of ACNP competencies, validated by the practitioners themselves in self-report surveys. There appears to be an evolving set of competencies. In addition, some of those listed below (Table 8.5) would only be acted on by ACNPs in related specialty areas (e.g., lumbar puncture).

These competencies are congruent with the role profiles described by Kleinpell (1997). Significant differences among the frequencies of specific items reflect those differences inherent within the choices that individual ACNPs make in how they choose to practice. For example, procedures reported as occurring most frequently in that study included giving nursing inservices and initiating quality assurance studies. These are reflective of the integrative role of the ACNP, drawing on nursing values, nursing departmental concerns, and activities designed for clinical nurse specialists and staff educators. Some ACNPs make their role

TABLE 8.3 Performance Description

Title: Nurse Practitioner, Acute Care (ACNP)
Department: Nursing
Purpose: Acute Care Nurse Practitioners (ACNP) are principal providers of care for acutely and/or critically ill patients. ACNPs are advanced practice nurses who provide a unique combination of advanced nursing and medical services for individuals and their families. ACNPs address the full range of health and illness services within their specialty area(s).

Emphasizing their clinical decision making skills, ACNPs:

- provide case management for a select group of patients in collaboration with the attending MD
- perform a comprehensive health assessment
- formulate diagnoses, and identify problems and health risk profiles
- perform, order and/or interpret diagnostic studies within scope of practice
- plan and implement therapeutic regimens which include both nursing and medical management strategies (including prescription of medications)
- initiate referrals and consultations with other advanced practice nurses, physicians and support services
- monitor and evaluate patient outcomes

Responsible to: Division Director of the units in collaboration with the Medical Director. In NICU, Manager of the Practitioner Program.

Resource to: Staff, Residents and students as appropriate.

The Acute Care Nurse Practitioner (ACNP) demonstrates the following behaviors:

1. Management and Coordination of Patient Care
   Summary Behavior: ACNPs provide care for acutely and/or critically ill patients. Their scope of practice includes both advanced nursing and medical components. ACNPs assume direct accountability for managing the care of a select group of patients.

Major Performance Responsibilities	Performance Standards	How Evaluated
1.1 Develops and implements a plan of care in collaboration with the family, physician, staff nurse, and other members of the health care team which incorporates acute care needs, health care	1.1.1 Collaborates with physicians, nurses, and other health disciplines to develop a comprehensive plan of care.	Self-reporting Report of Physicians, Nurse Manager, CNS, and Nursing Staff.

TABLE 8.3 *Continued*

Major Performance Responsibilities	Performance Standards	How Evaluated
maintenance, discharge, and follow up care.		
	1.1.2 Uses standards of care and current research in coordinating care to achieve desired patient outcomes.	As above
	1.1.3 Implements diagnostic and therapeutic interventions on a timely basis.	As above
	1.1.4 Evaluates physiological and behavioral responses to interventions for revision of management plan.	As above

2. Clinical Practice
Summary Behavior: Demonstrates the ability to make sound clinical assessments and to institute safe and efficacious routine and emergency care within the structure of a collaborative health care team.

Major Performance Responsibilities	Performance Standards	How Evaluated
2.1 Assessment/Planning: Gathers pertinent information systematically and skillfully from all sources: history, diagnostic tests, comprehensive physical examination, behavioral and developmental assessments.	2.1.1 Performs thorough and accurate health assessments, including history and physical.	Self-reporting Report of superordinates
	2.1.2 Differentiates normal and abnormal variations for all body systems.	As above
	2.1.3 Develops problem lists with associated differential diagnosis.	As above
	2.1.4 Incorporates available lab and imaging data into the plan of care.	As above

Continued

TABLE 8.3 *Continued*

Major Performance Responsibilities	Performance Standards	How Evaluated
	2.1.5 Identifies educational needs of the family and assists with teaching.	As above
	2.1.6 Alters plan of care as new data becomes available.	As above
	2.1.7 Presents patients in an organized manner on rounds which reflects thorough pre-round preparation.	Report of Physicians and Peers
2.2 Interventions: Provides therapeutic interventions which are selected/designed to incorporate knowledge of assessments, programs, goals and orders in the mode of action most likely to produce optimal outcome.	2.2.1 Establishes appropriate priorities of care.	Self Reporting Report of Physicians, Peers Report of Superordinate
	2.2.2 Appropriately orders, performs and interprets diagnostic tests.	As above
	2.2.3 Plans and implements appropriate pharmacologic therapies.	As above
	2.2.4 Accurately and appropriately performs routine diagnostic and therapeutic techniques according to established protocol and current standards for nurse practitioner practice.	As above
	2.2.5 Initiates referrals based on patient/family needs.	As above

TABLE 8.3 *Continued*

Major Performance Responsibilities	Performance Standards	How Evaluated
	2.2.6 Seeks appropriate consultation dependent upon patient health care needs.	As above
	2.2.7 Communicates with family regarding the changing health care needs of the patient.	As above
2.3 Evaluation: Bases evaluation on patient outcomes, revising practice to improve outcomes as needed.	2.3.1 Evaluates physiological and behavioral responses to interventions for revision of management plan.	Report of Superordinate Report of Physicians, Peers Self Reporting
	2.3.2 Participates in the systematic review of patient records, protocols, and treatment plans to determine the effectiveness in meeting established standards of care.	As above
	2.3.3 Participates in the development, review, and evaluation of nurse practitioner practice protocols.	As above
	2.3.4 Participates in self and peer evaluation to improve quality care.	As above

3. Education

Summary Behavior: Collaborates with the Nursing Manager and/or Clinical Nurse Specialist to support the educational needs of the nursing staff through behaviors consistent with an understanding of adult learning theory.

Continued

TABLE 8.3 *Continued*

Major Performance Responsibilities	Performance Standards	How Evaluated
3.1 Collaborates with the Nurse Manager and/or CNS to deliver educational support to the staff.	3.1.1 Participates in educational programs available to the nursing staff.	Self-reporting Report of Nurse Manager and/or CNS
	3.1.2 Supports educational directives/needs through informal bedside teaching based on accepted standards and available research.	Self-reporting Report of Physicians, Nurse Manager, CNS, and nursing staff
3.2 Facilitates the educational process of students affiliated with approved institutions.	3.2.1 Serves as a preceptor to students as appropriate.	Self-reporting Report of students

4. Consultation
Summary Behavior: Serves as a clinical consultant to peers, students, nursing staff, and house staff.

Major Performance Responsibilities	Performance Standards	How Evaluated
4.1 Provides clinical consultation to staff and to community agencies as requested.	4.1.1 Provides clinical consultation or provides referral information upon request.	Self-reporting Report of nursing, multidisciplinary house staff, and from community agencies.
	4.1.2 Bases consultation response on accepted standards and protocols and current research.	Self-reporting Report of superordinates Report of nursing, multidisciplinary, house staff, and from community agencies

5. Research
Summary Behavior: Supports research activities within the department and incorporates research data into practice within the structure of a collaborative multi-disciplinary team.

TABLE 8.3 *Continued*

Major Performance Responsibilities	Performance Standards	How Evaluated
5.1 Supports research activities within the unit.	5.1.1 Adheres to research protocols.	Self-reporting Report of superordinates Report of primary investigators
	5.1.2 Incorporates research data into practice as appropriate.	As above

6. Professional Development/Behaviors

Summary Behavior: Practices ethical behaviors which demonstrate professional commitment and responsibility to staff, patients, and families. Accepts responsibility and accountability for continued development of clinical skills and professional growth. Serves as a role model to other staff.

Major Performance Responsibilities	Performance Standards	How Evaluated
6.1 Demonstrates self-direction in professional goal setting	6.1.1 Participates in professional organizations.	Self-reporting
	6.1.2 Attends mandatory educational offerings.	Self-reporting Audit educational file
	6.1.3 Attends available medical, nursing and specialty in-house educational offerings.	As above Report of superordinates
	6.1.4 Keeps abreast of new developments in Clinical Specialty area.	Self-reporting Report of superordinates
	6.1.5 Develops plan for attaining professional performance goals on annual basis.	Self-reporting Shares written goals at evaluation
	6.1.6 Independently evaluates progress in meeting performance objectives and goals.	Completes self-evaluation and is prepared to discuss at evaluation

Continued

TABLE 8.3 *Continued*

Major Performance Responsibilities	Performance Standards	How Evaluated
	6.1.7 Abides by protocols and the Standards of the Department of Nursing and Medicine.	Self-reporting Report of superordinates
6.2 Contributes to cohesiveness of unit and facilitates intergroup functioning/cooperation.	6.2.1 Participates in active problem solving for unit and interdepartmental issues.	As above Documented attendance at staff meetings and other appropriate, unit/department meetings.
6.2.2	Demonstrates understanding of principles of group dynamics, change theory, conflict resolution, and team building.	Self-reporting Report of superordinates Report of peers, medical, and nursing staff
	6.2.3 Demonstrates awareness of professional responsibility as role model to peers and nursing staff.	As above
6.3 Functions according to the philosophies and objectives of the Departments of Medicine and Nursing and within Hospital policy.	6.3.1 States policies correctly to families, professional staff members, and other employees.	Superordinate and peer reports
6.4 Participants in unit QA/QI activities.	6.4.1 Facilitates/participates in disciplines specific and multidisciplinary QA/QI activities.	Self-report, documentation Superordinate report QA/QI report
6.5 Knowledgeable of relevant JCAHO standards.	6.5.1 Incorporates knowledge of JCAHO standards into clinical practice.	Self-report, documentation Superordinate report

TABLE 8.3 *Continued*

6. Requirements

6.1 *Experience*:
One year experience as a Nurse Practitioner in area of Clinical Specialty preferred.

6.2 *Education*:
Masters degree in nursing preferred. Successful completion of Nurse Practitioner Program. National certification as a Nurse Practitioner required for experienced Nurse Practitioners. New Practitioners are required to obtain national certification as soon as they meet the requirements for application.

6.3 *Licensure*:
Current RN licensure in Connecticut. Subsequent APRN licensure in Connecticut.

6.4 *Credentialing*:
After completing APRN licensure must attain credentialing through the Nursing Professional Practice Council in collaboration with the John Dempsey Hospital Medical Board.

6.5 *Contacts*:
Attending and residency physicians; physicians and nursing staff from regional allied/affiliated hospitals; consulting attending physicians; community health team members; nursing staff across multiple units; medication nursing and students; Clinic personnel; patient's immediate and extended family members; and patients.

6.6 *Variables*:
Rotation of shifts covering days and nights; shift duration between 8 and 16 hours, with the potential of extension of hours beyond scheduled shift time. Includes weekends and holidays.

6.7 *Work Characteristics*:
Frequent physical demands which include walking, standing, lifting, pulling, pushing, stooping and stretching. Potential exposure to infection risk. Frequent exposure to a highly pressured and rapidly changing environment.

6.8 *Pay Grade*:
UHPC 6

6.9 *Approved*:
January, 1994

Note. From The University of Connecticut Health Center, John Dempsey Hospital, Farmington, CT. Reprinted with permission.

operational to include large components of the consultative or educative function; others use components that are more involved with provision of direct patient care. Further elaboration of the collaborative nature of the ACNP role is needed, so that realistic expectations and evaluation of this practitioner may occur.

TABLE 8.4 ACNP Evaluation Survey Form: Nurse Colleagues

Items common to all nurses surveyed

1. The ANCP recognizes changes in clinical status of patients and responds appropriately to those changes.
2. The ACNP recognizes and responds appropriately to emergency situations.
3. The ACNP uses an effective communication style with other nurses.
4. The ACNP uses an effective communication style with other members of the health care team.

Items shared by staff nurses and clinical nurse specialists

5. I feel comfortable when the ACNP is the first-line practitioner for a patient.
6. I feel comfortable when the ANCP is the first-line practitioner for a critically ill patient.
7. I believe that the ACNP is effective in planning the day-to-day care and treatment goals for the patients.
8. The ACNP facilitates and enhances my communication with patients and families.
9. I feel that the ACNP offers unique clinical support and education as compared with other practitioners.

Item for clinical nurse specialist

10. I believe that the ACNP role compromises my influence as a clinical nurse specialist.

Items for nurse managers

11. I find the ACNP is a resource to me as a nurse manager.
12. I feel the staff is receptive to the role of the ACNP.
13. I believe that the ACNP role compromises my authority as a nurse manager.
14. I think it is possible in the future to run the unit effectively using only nonphysicians as first-line practitioners.

FUTURE DIRECTIONS FOR ACUTE CARE NURSE PRACTITIONER EVALUATION

Although the work to date is commendable, much still needs to be done. The large number of factors or variables to be studied have been arranged here according to the traditional evaluation pathways of structure, process, and outcomes.

Structure Evaluation Pathways

Structure has frequently been used as the beginning point for developing evaluation schemes. Structure refers to both the health care environment, setting and organization— and the characteristics of the health care providers—their number, education, and demographics (Fink, 1993). The

TABLE 8.5 Competencies for ACNPs

Demonstrates knowledge of advanced pathophysiology in the following areas:
- neurology
- cardiology
- pulmonary concerns
- renal concerns
- endocrinology
- gastrointestinal concerns
- fluid balance
- acid/base balance

Completes a health history

Conducts a partial or complete physical exam

Demonstrates ability to appropriately order and interpret the following:
- arterial blood gases
- venous blood analyses
- cardiac enzymes
- coagulation measures
- liver function tests
- urinalysis/culture
- x-rays—abdominal/chest/routine
- 12-lead EKG

Demonstrates technical skill with the following procedures:

Cardiovascular:	Arterial puncture/cannulation/line removal
	IAPB management
	Pulmonary artery catheter: management/removal/insertion
	Resuscitation management
	Vasoactive drugs: initiation/management
Pulmonary:	Airway management
	Endotracheal tubes: insertion/management/removal
	Oxygen devices
	Chest tube-insertion/management/removal
	Thoracentesis
	Ventilator management: initiation/maintenance/weaning parameters
Gastrointestinal:	Nasogastric/intestinal tube: insertion/removal
	G-tube: re-insertion/management/removal
	Paracentesis
	Nutritional therapies: initiation/maintenance
Neurological:	Lumbar puncture
Renal:	Peritoneal dialysis: management/removal of catheter
	Bladder: suprapubic aspiration
Miscellaneous:	Institutes blood component therapies
	Administration of intradermal tests
	Cutaneous suturing
	Venous catheter insertion/management: central/peripheral/cut down

Continued

TABLE 8.5 *Continued*

Wounds: management/debridement/packing
Apply local anesthesia
Perform cultures
Collaborates with other care providers to facilitate positive patient outcomes.
Consultations: initiation
Discharge planning: initiation

assumption with structure evaluation is that when the structural elements are positive, the outcomes will also be positive. This may not necessarily be the case, however. Other structural factors include job descriptions, performance evaluation procedures, reporting structures, communication patterns, resources, inclusion in relevant organization groups and activities, and credentialing requirements. Despite doubts as to the outcome it is imperative that structural elements support the objective, in this case, successful practice for ACNPs.

Setting

The organization where the ACNP is located may be an institution or a professional group. The health-care setting may be public or private; fee-for-service or global fee scales and managed care may dominate. Private, fee-for-service arrangements with medical specialty groups provide ease for the discernment of discreet activities attributable to the ACNP if the coding allows for these distinctions. Publicly funded settings are more likely to employ a cadre of providers, and providing care is often team based, resulting in global billing. Outcomes attributable to any individual ACNP or group of ACNPs is confounded by the team approach. Aspects of cost effectiveness are buried within complicated formulas for determining bed rates and staff salaries. Clinical outcomes are also difficult to trace because so many provider types are integrated in the patient care delivery scheme.

The organization may employ only one ACNP or many. The practitioner may be of one subspecialty (e.g., cardiology), or several may be deployed on a single unit (intensive care). Perhaps the institution considers all practitioners as one group regardless of specialty, thus joining those whose specialties encompass out of hospital care (ambulatory clinics, employee health) with those who are strictly hospital unit-based. Any examination of institutional outcomes should take into consideration structural elements, such as the many types of practitioners potentially factored into outcome data. The number of the same type of practitioner may also steer outcomes. Practice patterns of a cohort of ACNPs with the luxury of cross coverage may not resemble that of a solitary, perhaps off-shift, practitioner. Overtime demands may compromise quality of care. Structural description should, therefore, include the relationships among the multiple practitioners included in any outcome evaluation.

Reporting

Another aspect of the setting is the organizational structure as it applies to reporting or hierarchical relationships. To whom do the ACNPs report? In situations in which the reporting is made to medical supervisors, the opportunity exists for losing some elements of the holistic nursing approach. Perhaps it is thought that the practitioners spend too much time with patients and families on nonclinical matters. ACNPs are also central to clinical instruction occurring on acute care units. The potential for conflicting loyalties is also present. With a variety of clinical student types present in need of teaching, the medical supervisors may place increased value on activities related to teaching medical students and less on other nursing students.

When the reporting structure is made to the nursing administrators, the problems cited above are minimized. Do all nursing supervisors who are not practitioners truly understand the demands of the practitioner world? Can clinical excellence be recognized? These troubling questions may give rise to dual reporting systems that mitigate some of the problems. Evaluation methods need to account for these differences.

Demographics

As mentioned before, the demographics of any focus group relates to structural evaluation. In the case of ACNPs, the nature and type of education should be noted. Were the ACNPs prepared within formal practitioner programs? Were the programs designed for the acute care environment or were they basically primary care programs with acute care specialty clinical requirements? In contrast, the ACNPs may have completed institutionally based training programs that were specifically designed to meet the needs of the host institution. By their very design, these programs would vary in length, focus, and quality. Transferability of skills and competencies may be called into question. These practitioners may or may not be eligible for certification. These items add to the data needed for broad structure evaluation.

Communication Patterns

With the recognition that communication is a specialty of its own, one may still see that formal and informal communication patterns exist within organizations. Much to the chagrin of the unknowing and uninitiated, the informal patterns are indeed powerful. At times they can be more powerful than the formal routes of exchange. Of interest then is the dialogue pattern that exists within a group of ACNPs and between ACNPs and other members of the care team. Evaluation questions to be asked include to whom the ACNP directs inquiries about patients, other staff, personal scheduling preferences, policies, procedures, complaints, and ethical decision making.

Another aspect of communication patterns is *access*: access to people, restricted information, committees, administrators, noontime conferences, grand rounds, and so on. This has implications for ACNP work scheduling. If the ACNP is covering patient care in the offshift time periods, access to elements of the organization is severely restricted.

Resources

As with any position, infrastructure support in the form of structural resources has a profound influence on outcomes and performance. Structural evaluation should account for clerical support, professional literature, computers, office space, space for personal belongings, and security and access to them all. Often the supports in place are shared among all team or unit members. For example, clerical staff in hospitals usually have responsibilities for patients that supersede nonpatient requests. Most hospitals also have health science libraries that are readily accessible. In situations in which ACNPs are employed outside of hospitals, the reverse may be true. Clerical staff serve the office, but libraries are on the hospital or health center campus. Differences pertain to space issues as well. Hospitals were designed for use in a different era of care delivery, and they reflect the needs that existed then. Space for conferences, quiet reflection, and team dialogue and rounds; computer access for a multitude of users; desk or writing space; and chart access are only a few of the challenges that greet care providers in most current acute care settings.

Organization Groups and Activities

The structural evaluation should account for formal and informal alliances and the position of the ACNP within the system. Standing committees often have a powerful influence over the usual and customary care practices within hospitals. To the extent that ACNPs are directing patient care, their voices should be represented in the entire spectrum of committees affecting patient care. Educational conferences, grand rounds, teaching rounds, unit meetings, specialty meetings, morbidity and mortality discussions, and departmental meetings are all requisite activities for ACNPs. Evaluations will determine whether or not these activities are occurring and why.

Credentialing Requirements

The structure and organization of ACNP credentialing is as important to the evaluation of the ACNP as it is to other professional staff members, for example, physicians, within the acute care setting. Advanced practice nurses within hospitals occupy a peculiar position vis-à-vis the credentialing process. Medical staffs appoint standing committees to analyze applicants' (usually MDs or DOs) credentials when requests for staff privileges are made. These committees comprise medical personnel who are able to make judgments concerning their colleagues' qualifications. Unfortunately, they are not qualified to make similar judgments concerning nurses and may be unable to discern the differences among the wide scope of nursing preparation. Yet, they are responsible for granting the privileges needed for ACNPs to function.

For this reason and to reinforce nursings' professional role in the ACNP, nursing professional practice boards have been established at some institutions to review applicants prior to the medical staff review. This situation can be likened to the earlier days of progress in nursing research. Research proposals dealing with nursing problems were often initially screened by a nursing research review panel prior to being submitted to the institutional review board. More recently, the composition of these boards has been rearranged to include representation from the nursing profession. System changes for the future may result in similar reconfiguration on the credentialing and privileging bodies of acute care institutions to include nurses in advanced practice.

Furthermore, because the role is so new, few standards have been proposed for credentialing ACNPs beyond the specialty practitioner certification offered jointly by the American Nurses' Credentialing Corporation with the American Association of Critical Care Nurses. Evaluation of the processes in place will assist with this development so that future graduates and employees will benefit from specific standard criteria.

Process Evaluation Pathways

Evaluation of the process focuses on activities. It examines the technical and human aspects of care provision by answering the question of what is done to and for patients (Fink, 1993). It is recommended that baseline data be collected in advance of this evaluation step whenever possible.

On the humanistic aspect one can examine the interpersonal skills of the ACNPs: communication style, collaboration, and consultation. Communication style reflects how ACNPs relate to the patients as well as all others pivotal to the care delivered: staff nurses, staff physicians, pharmacists, nutritionists, physician assistants, technicians, and others on the interdisciplinary team. Communication types include verbal, written, and electronic. Verbal communication can be measured by survey of opinion or direct observation. Chart review and examination of data stored in electronic systems provides a source of evaluation material for other patterns of communication. Anecdotal evidence reported by Shah et al. (1997) attests to the high quality of written chart data contributed by ACNPs.

Technical skills assigned to the domain of nurse practitioners vary by geography and institutions or the culture of the employing group. Evaluation should address the number and type of any procedures done over a fixed period of time. A simple check list such as the one shown in Table 8.6 can produce the needed information.

In addition to determining the number and type of procedures done, evaluation should include any errors or complications that may have occurred. Were these in the presence of senior ranked preceptors? Institutions vary in methods for dealing with the problems of provider-initiated complications. These vary from special patient care committees to quality assessment monitors and to morbidity and mortality rounds. The former common designation of "acceptable complication" has little meaning in current health care environments in view of the increasing presence of litigation. Scrupulous attention to provider-sourced variance is needed to prevent escalation of care delivery problems. Careful monitoring of these aspects of care is part of the technical evaluation.

Conceptual skill is also a component of the technical aspect of care but is more difficult to measure. This involves the ability of the practitioner to assimilate and synthesize patient data for adequate and comprehensive case presentation during rounds. Were the salient elements of the case presented along with the relationship of these elements to the problem and therapies indicated? What was the overall relationship to any action taken? What questions were asked, tests ordered, and notes recorded?

TABLE 8.6 Procedure Verification List

Procedure	Supervised Yes	Supervised Successfully	Alone Yes	Alone Successfully
Venipuncture				
Arterial puncture				
Arterial line cannulation				
Internal jugular line insertion				
Subclavian line insertion				
Femoral line insertion				
Pulmonary artery catheter removal				
Pulmonary artery catheter insertion				
Thoracotomy tube insertion				
Thoracentesis				
Dialysis catheter insertion				
Nasogastric tube insertion				
Lumbar puncture				
Electrocardiogram recording (12 lead)				
Removal of chest tubes				
Change central venous lines				
Adjustment of intra-aortic counterpulsation devices				
Cardiopulmonary resuscitation				
Participant				
"Run the code" (in charge)				
Endotracheal intubation				
Administration of intradermal skin tests				
Suturing minor lacerations				
Removal of staples				
Cleanse/debride wound				

Finally, the actual process of care should be addressed. Items to be included are the number of hours worked, the number of cases being covered by an individual or the team, the morbidity of the case load, and the time spent in rounds.

Outcomes Evaluation Pathways

As Hegyvary (1991) so aptly described, defining and measuring outcomes of care is exceedingly complex and challenging. There is widespread agreement, however, that outcomes evaluation must continue to receive the highest priority attention. Hegyvary (1991) identified five issues related to the evaluation of patient care outcomes:

1. The definition of outcomes varies widely by author and may include Lohr's classic definition of death, disease, disability, discomfort, and dissatisfaction. Specific quantitative measures of health and quality care as well as affective variables such as quality of life, social functioning, and general well-being are also of importance. To date there is no standard agreement on how to categorize outcomes measures or what should be included in each category.

2. The timing of outcome evaluation can greatly affect the findings. In many cases, a repeated measures design will better capture the true results of a program or intervention since life and health are not linear concepts but continuous processes.

3. Several different levels of analysis are of interest to various researchers, including individual, groups (including disease management), and societal (which would necessarily need to include a cost-benefit analysis) outcomes. These different levels of analysis require different variables and approaches, all of which must be taken into account when designing an outcome evaluation.

4. Attribution, or the determination of causal variables, is a particular challenge to outcomes researchers. In many cases, multiple factors are responsible for the outcomes achieved. Most evaluation schema do not provide for the scientific rigor required to establish causality or the relative contribution of several variables, yet, that is frequently the interpretation derived from the evaluation data presented.

5. The existence or availability of an appropriate comparative database is a continuing problem for most evaluators and researchers. Although there has been a significant increase in the amount of data available for many investigations, the lack of standardized definitions and measures continues to inhibit the ability to access important information.

Jones (1993) presented a concise overview of the approaches and issues influencing outcomes across hospitals, which are the primary setting for ACNP practice. Macrolevel approaches include

- *Direct standardization*: attempts to isolate the effects of hospital care on patient outcomes. It is not possible to measure changing health status with existing databases, however. The alternative application of measuring variations in the rates of adverse complications across hospitals assumes that patient outcomes are better in hospitals, where there are fewer adverse events.

- *Meta-analysis*: systematically combines the results from several studies. Although valuable, the meta-analysis is often impractical because the number of studies similar enough to evaluate are insufficient. Additionally, the meta-analysis does not focus on differences between settings or providers, which contribute substantially to assessing patient outcomes related to the ACNP role.
- *Small area analysis*: population-based studies that use assumptions regarding utilization rates as reflections of quality, for example, hospital admissions, provider visits, and a number of surgical procedures such as hysterectomy and hernia repair, and so on. Difficulty in establishing clear standards for comparing utilization rates are a major deficit to this approach.
- *Indirect standardization*: (the most common approach) is the study of outcomes at the hospital or system level, with adjustments made for the types of patients treated (case mix and severity of illness adjustments along with other quantifiable variations).

The evaluation of patient outcomes is a challenging endeavor. Numerous contributory factors are inherent in virtually every evaluation study, including the wide variation in health professionals who provide care, the severity and course of the patient's illness, and the structure of and resources available to deliver care.

Ingersoll (1995) summarized evaluation of the advanced practice nurse role in acute and specialty care. Considerations that must be emphasized include the need to evaluate both individual ACNP performance and overall role contributions to systems improvement, compliance with regulatory requirements, and enhancement of perceptions of a variety of customers, including patients. In this regard, it becomes essential to avoid simply comparing ACNPs with medical residents or attending physicians. Although there is considerable role overlap in the provision of direct patient care, the related roles of these groups differ dramatically. As Ingersoll (1995) notes,

> The medical resident, as student, is assessed primarily for proficiency and accuracy of task performance, whereas the ACNP [as practitioner] is evaluated for task performance as well as the coordination of care delivery, ability to facilitate smooth patient progress throughout the health care

TABLE 8.7 Framework for Patient Outcomes Evaluation

	Patients/SOs	MDs/RNs	Payors
Clinical	Physiological status Pathophysiological outcomes Psychosocial well-being	Physiological status Pathophysiological outcomes Psychosocial well-being Morbidity & mortality	Health status Morbidity & mortality Referrals & consultations
Functional	Physical functional abilities Ability to fulfill social role Time lost to health problems	Physical functional abilities Ability to fulfill social role Time lost to health problems	Physical functional abilities Return to work
Perceptual	Satisfaction with clinical, functional, and financial outcomes Satisfaction with care Knowledge for self-care	Patient satisfaction with outcomes Patient satisfaction with process of care Patient knowledge Health professional collaboration and communication Health professional knowledge and skills	Patient satisfaction Patient knowledge Communication with payors
Financial	Overall charges/costs Amounts not covered by payor	Charges/cost of care LOS Postdischarge resource needs Health professional productivity/salary	Charges/cost of care LOS Postdischarge resource needs Continuity/coordination as affect costs

system, interpersonal interactions with care providers and patients or families, and availability when needed. (p. 28)

Two conceptual works can be used to provide a framework for exploring outcomes assessment related to ACNPs. First, Hegyvary (1991) suggested four categories of outcomes: clinical, functional, perceptual, and financial, which allow for the organization of significant outcome measures. Clinical outcomes include patient responses to medical and nursing interventions. Specific indicators would be developed for various situations and might incorporate the health status of patients related to their disease and pathophysiological conditions, symptom management, mortality and morbidity, and other clinical elements used to track improvement or progression of a given disease entity. Functional outcomes relate to maintenance or improvement of physical functioning and patients' ability to perform in the various social roles occupied, including caring for self, family roles and interaction, work, and social activities. Perceptual outcomes relate to patient satisfaction with outcomes, care received, and providers. Finally, financial outcomes analyze relationships between outcomes in the other areas and resources consumed to achieve those outcomes.

The second conceptual element is the stakcholder model of evaluation. Although patients remain the center of focus, there are numerous other important stakeholders who would prudently be incorporated into a comprehensive outcomes evaluation framework. For the purposes of organizing the approach to ACNP outcomes evaluation, the following stakeholder perspectives will be addressed: patients and significant others, physicians and nurses, and payors. Table 8.7 is a grid that depicts the combination of outcomes categories with key stakeholders and contains the priority variables for each cell of the grid. Some variables could easily be considered in multiple cells; in these cases, discussion occurs only once under the primary assignment. The variables are further defined in the following sections.

Clinical Outcomes

Patients are most interested in the correct diagnosis and selection of interventions and treatment for their health problems, along with their psychosocial well-being. Physicians and nurses are similarly interested in these variables and in addition evaluate physiological status, pathophysiological changes, and morbidity and mortality. Payors are most interested in health status, morbidity and mortality, and the use of referrals and consultation.

The evaluation of clinical outcomes is increasingly popular, especially incorporating the assessment of those who serve as the primary responsible coordinator and deliverer of care, for example, ACNPs. Unfortunately, only a handful of studies that specifically evaluate the clinical outcomes of ACNP patients have been reported to date.

Functional Outcomes

Patients' priorities relate to changing their ability to perform various physical activities and the amount of time spent on dealing with health issues. Physicians, nurses, and payors have similar interests in the area of functional outcomes, although payors also evaluate patient ability to return to productive employment as an important measure.

Perceptual Outcomes

The premier variable in this category for all stakeholders is overall patient satisfaction, with outcomes in the other categories: clinical, functional, and financial. In addition, patients need to have appropriate knowledge of their condition and treatment to effectively care for themselves. Physicians and nurses are also interested in perceived collaboration and in communication among providers with major responsibility for patient care. Health professionals also have opinions about the knowledge and skills of their colleagues, particularly among roles that can provide similar services, such as nurse practitioners and physicians. Last, payors assess the ease and accuracy of communication and information provided by various professionals and institutions.

Financial Outcomes

The general consideration in this category is the relationship of resources consumed to outcomes achieved. Length of stay is of interest to all stakeholders, since the number of days of inpatient care is directly related to the overall resource consumption and subsequent cost of an episode of care. For patients, the concerns relate to overall costs of care and particularly those costs not covered by their payor. Nurses and physicians are increasingly cognizant of the costs of care, from both providing service in the acute care setting and the subsequent need for postdischarge support. Payors usually include a measure of the continuity and coordination of care, since these are also related to resource usage.

Acute Care Nurse Practitioner Outcomes Studies

Few outcomes studies that specifically evaluate the role of the ACNP have been reported. Ingersoll (1995) reported that only one formal evaluation of the ACNP role was found (Spisso, O'Callaghan, & McKennan, 1990). This study evaluated the contributions of trauma nurse practitioners in a regional trauma center. The findings indicated that the addition of ACNPs to the trauma service reduced patient length of stay (LOS), improved the quality of care, and increased patient satisfaction.

As discussed earlier, recently published studies have focused on aspects of the ACNP role (Kleinpell, 1997; Shah et al., 1997). Shah et al. (1997), in addition to incorporating the performance review information referenced earlier, sought to document perceptual outcome data from a variety of stakeholders. The identified stakeholders were physicians, nurse administrators, clinical nurse specialists, nurse managers, and staff nurses in the areas of critical skills, patient management and coordination, collaboration and communication with staff, and unique contributions of the ACNPs to the care environment. The previously cited survey by Kleinpell (1997) established the common role elements of a substantial number of ACNPs across numerous settings.

If one broadens the evaluation focus to advanced practice nurses, the meta-analysis previously mentioned (Brown & Grimes, 1993) provides the most comprehensive analysis and interpretation of available data. Knauss, Felten, Burton, Fobes, and Davis (1997) reported that primary nurse practitioners working in the acute care setting spent 39% of their time in direct patient care with excellent patient satisfaction. Without exception, studies of advanced practice nurses have shown that nurse practitioners provide care equivalent to or superior to that of physicians (Mundinger, 1993). Many more data related to all aspects of outcomes for evaluating ACNP practice are needed.

SUMMARY

The intent of this chapter has been to describe the conceptual and practical elements for the evaluation of ACNPs. Because this is a relatively new professional role and specific role functions may overlap those already existing within the health care system, it is a complex process. The evaluation of ACNPs suffers from the same challenges that pertain to most program or role evaluation. Activities do not occur in a vacuum, and discreet behaviors or outcomes are unavoidably confounded by other variables.

Many similarities exist between the ACNP role development story and the original nurse practitioner movement. There is evidence in the literature showing beginning efforts in delineating role functions and perceptions of various stakeholders within the health-care system.

Program evaluation may be organized in multiple forms: by program characteristics and merits or by use of several frameworks, such as the stakeholder framework or the structure-process-outcome framework. A clearly defined plan with identified goals and objectives using a specific framework is the recommended starting point.

Recent attention to outcomes has provoked scholarly discourse regarding how best to achieve the goal of measuring outcomes. Hegyvary's (1991) recommendation of using four broad conceptual categories can be combined with elements of the stakeholder model to serve as a departure point for an evaluation project.

Although there are many valid and useful elements related to ACNP practice to examine, the future focus of ACNP evaluation must be on patient outcomes in the domains previously described (clinical, functional, perceptual, and financial) rather than on structure, process, or sociological factors. As more ACNPs gain experience in managing groups of patients and the quality and availability of patient data improve, the stage should be set for extensive documentation of care outcomes.

REFERENCES

Bandura, A. (1977). Self-efficacy: Toward a unifying theory of behavioral change. *Psychology Review, 84,* 191–215.

Bernal, H., & Froman, R. (1987). The confidence of community health nurses in caring for ethnically diverse populations. *Image: Journal of Nursing Scholarship, 19*(4), 201–203.

Brown, S.A., & Grimes, D.E. (1993). *Nurse practitioners and certified nurse-midwives: A meta-analysis of studies on nurses in primary care roles.* Washington, DC: American Nursing Publishing.

Fink, A. (1993). *Evaluation fundamentals.* Newbury Park, CA: Sage.

Froman, R., & Owen, S.V. (1991). High school students' perceived self-efficacy in physical and mental health. *Journal of Adolescent Research, 6*(2), 181–196.

Hegyvary, S.T. (1991). Issues in outcomes research. *Journal of Nursing Quality Assurance, 5*(2), 1–6.

Ingersoll, G.L. (1995). Evaluation of the advanced practice nurse role in acute and specialty care. *Critical Care Clinics of North America, 7*(1), 25–33.

Johnson, J.H., & Olesinski, N. (1995). Program evaluation. *Journal of Nursing Administration, 25*(1), 53–60.

Jones, K.R. (1993). Outcomes analysis: Methods and issues. *Nursing Economics, 11*(3), 145–152.

Kleinpell, R.M. (1997). Acute care nurse practitioners: roles and practice profiles. *AACN Clinical Issues, 8*(1), 156–162.

Knauss, V.L., Felten, S., Burton, S., Fobes, P., & Davis, K. (1997). The use of nurse practitioners in the acute care setting. *Journal of Nursing Administration,* 27(2), 20–27.

Mallison, M.B. (1993). Nurses as house staff. *American Journal of Nursing, 93*(3), 7.

Mundinger, M. (1993). Advanced practice nursing—good medicine for physicians. *New England Journal of Medicine, 330,* 211.

Rossi, P., & Freeman, H. (1993). *Evaluation: a systematic approach.* Newbury Park, CA: Sage.

Shah, H.S., Bruttomesso, K.A., Taylor Sullivan, D., & Lattanzio, J. (1997). An evaluation of the role and practices of the acute care nurse practitioner. *AACN Clinical Issues, 8*(1), 147–155.

Silver, H.K., Ford, L.C., & Day, L.R. (1968). The pediatric nurse practitioner program. *American Journal of Nursing, 68* (3), 822–824.

Silver, H.K., & McAtee, P. (1988). Should nurses substitute for house staff? *American Journal of Nursing, 88*(12), 1671–1673.

Spisso, J., O'Callaghan, C., & McKennan, M. (1990). Improved quality of care and reduction of house staff workload using trauma nurse practitioners. *Journal of Trauma, 30,* 660.

9

The Acute Care Nurse Practitioner in the Emergency Department Setting

Frank L. Cole and Janine M. Catalano*

The role of the acute care nurse practitioner (ACNP) in the emergency department (ED) setting is a multifaceted and challenging one. This chapter explores issues related to the practice of the ACNP in the ED. An overview of the development of emergency services and components of the ED are described. Results from a national study of users of emergency services are provided to highlight conditions the ACNP will most likely encounter in the ED setting. The role of the ACNP in the ED is discussed in terms of the various aspects of practice in this setting.

HISTORY OF EMERGENCY SERVICES

Following World War II and the Depression, there was a severe shortage of hospitals. In 1946, Congress enacted the Hospital Survey and Construction Act, more commonly known as the Hill-Burton Act. The initial emphasis of this act was on the construction of new hospitals; later more emphasis was placed on the modernization of existing facilities. Through the Hill-Burton Act, many of the nation's EDs were established and

*The first author would like to acknowledge the financial assistance of the Department of Health & Human Services, Health Resources and Services Administration, Bureau of Health Professions, Division of Nursing, Advanced Nurse Education Grant #1-023-NU-01193-01.

mandated to provide 24-hour emergency care to all clients (Haglund & Dowling, 1993). According to Kovner (1995), the vast majority of hospitals in the United States have EDs. EDs provide services to persons with a variety of illnesses ranging from minor to life threatening and often serve as a primary source of admissions to the hospital. Yet, the advent and growth of these departments has taken more than 50 years.

The inadequacy of emergency medical services (EMS) in the United States was highlighted when the National Research Council of the National Academy of Science published its report on the status of emergency care in 1966. The report, Accidental Death and Disability: The Neglected Disease of Modern Society, was prepared by the committees on trauma, shock, and anesthesia (National Academy of Sciences, 1996). Among other problems, this report identified that few individuals in EMS were trained in childbirth or cardiopulmonary resuscitation or other life-saving procedures. Moreover, most people assume that every ED can provide a full range of services from nonurgent care to massive trauma care; not every hospital had the personnel or equipment to provide a full range of services, however. The National Academy of Science (1966) recommended that hospital EDs be categorized based on physical availability, nursing staff, equipment, and personnel necessary to provide care.

The impetus for change in emergency services was provided through two acts. The first was when the National Highway Transportation Safety Act of 1966 authorized the Department of Transportation to improve EMS, especially ambulance services and development of prehospital personnel. The second was when Emergency Medicine was recognized by the American Board of Medical Specialists as the 23rd medical specialty in 1979 (MacPhail, 1992). Once recognized as a specialty, research and better ways of caring for emergency patients developed.

EDs were once staffed predominantly by interns who relied on residents for assistance with complicated cases. Currently, EDs tend to be staffed by physicians who have completed their postgraduate training; however, it is preferable to staff the ED with physicians who have completed an accredited emergency medicine residency program and are board certified in Emergency Medicine.

HISTORY OF EMERGENCY NURSE PRACTITIONERS

Midlevel providers are not uncommon in emergency services. The first emergency nurse practitioner programs existed in the late 1970s (Hardy, 1978; Hayden, Davies, & Clore, 1982). These programs educated nurses to provide health care services in EDs but were short lived. Since that time, nurse practitioners who provided emergency services have been educated in adult, family, and pediatric programs. These programs, however, are focused on primary care and do not provide the skills or knowledge needed to care for individuals with urgent or emergent conditions. Recently, the ACNP programs have provided experiences for individuals interested in emergency services. In 1994 the School of Nursing at the University of Texas-Houston implemented an emergency nurse practitioner (ENP) program that can be completed in 21 months of full-time study. This ENP program provides the skill and knowledge to provide health care in emergency services. In addition to the core courses of nursing theory, research, statistics, and research synthesis, students must successfully complete advanced pharmacology; physical examination and differential diagnosis (45 lab hours of practice); advanced pathophysiology; advanced practice in nursing: economics and management of health care systems; and advanced practice in nursing: primary prevention in individuals, families, and communities (45 hours of clinical practice). Courses specific to the ENP include diagnostic tests and procedures for emergency nurse practitioners and ACNPs (45 hours of lab experience); acute symptoms management (90 hours of clinical); treatment of health deviations in emergency care I (90 hours of clinical); treatment of health deviations in emergency care II (90 hours of clinical); and advanced clinical practice: nurse practitioner role and preceptorship—emergency and ambulatory care (400 hours of clinical). The above courses that are specific to the ENP provide knowledge and experience with diagnostic and therapeutic skills, outlined in Table 9.1, as well as assessing, diagnosing, and treating specific nonurgent to life-threatening conditions.

COMPONENTS OF THE EMERGENCY DEPARTMENT

The emergency department is an organized and coordinated system that consists of several components. The ACNP must be familiar with the components of the ED to understand the functioning of the total department. Moreover, the ACNP may be employed to provide services within one specific component or within multiple components. Each different area requires specialized competencies as well as versatility in commu-

TABLE 9.1 Diagnostic and Therapeutic Skills For Emergency Care

Incision/drainage of abscesses
Chest tube insertion
Needle decompression of the chest
Cricothyrotomy/tracheostomy
Endotracheal intubation/airway management
Suturing of lacerations and wounds
Nerve blocks
12-Lead electrocardiogram interpretation
Radiograph interpretation
Laboratory test interpretation
Microscopy of blood, urine, and other body fluids
Splinting of injuries/stabilization of fractures
Lumbar punctures
Needle aspiration of joints
Venisection/central vascular access devices
Thoracentesis

nicating with clients and their families. In most EDs, all staff are required to be competent in the care of clients across the life span from the moment of birth to death. Additionally, most EDs require that personnel, including nurse practitioners, physician assistants, physicians, nurses, and other ancillary staff, be flexible and able to staff any area of the ED at any time. Although components and responsibilities of the ACNP may vary among facilities, the following provides a brief overview of typical ED components and the services provided.

Prehospital

Prehospital services are those services provided before the person arrives in the ED. These services are often referred to as being provided "in the field." Prehospital services may be provided by city or county EMS, by a private ambulance company, or by a hospital-based EMS. Upon arrival at the ED, prehospital providers transfer care of a person to the ED personnel.

The ACNP may be required to fulfill a variety of functions related to prehospital care. Some EDs provide "medical control" for area EMS or for their own hospital-based EMS. The ACNP may be required to direct

EMS personnel, usually emergency medical technicians (EMTs) or paramedics (EMT-Ps), by radio or other communications device in their care of the client in the field. Although some EMS personnel are employed primarily in EMS, many others are volunteers who infrequently answer calls, especially calls to complex situations. Directions may range from administration of medications to permission to perform potentially life-saving procedures such as tracheoesophageal intubation, cricothyrotomy, or chest decompression. In the case of EMS personnel who respond infrequently to complex calls, the ACNP must be able to provide detailed instructions to the EMS provider performing a low-frequency, high-skill procedure.

Other facilities, usually those with hospital-based EMS, may require the ACNP to accompany the EMTs, EMT-Ps, or registered nurses (RNs), or a combination of these, to the scene of the emergency. Transportation to the scene may be by ground (conventional ambulances) or air. Air transportation is described as being by rotor or fixed wing, with rotor representing a helicopter and fixed wing denoting a plane. In this situation the ACNP generally is in charge of the team and may or may not have communication with a more experienced provider for consultation. The ACNP may also be required to accompany critical or unstable patients when they are transferred to a facility providing a higher level of care or to pick up unstable clients from outlying facilities. Again, this transportation may be by ground in an ambulance or by air. Regardless of the reason for transport, the ACNP who is required to participate in any sort of air transport must receive specialized training in air safety and care of the patient during air transfer.

The ACNP must cultivate and maintain good working relationships with all EMS personnel who transport clients to the ACNP's facility. Often, the EMS personnel are familiar with those clients they transport frequently and are able to provide valuable information that may otherwise be difficult to obtain. The EMS personnel may also be perceived by the client or family as someone with whom they can share information that they might neglect to tell the ACNP. Finally, in many communities where more than one facility is available, the EMS personnel transporting the patient decide which patient will be transported to which facility. These decisions are often based on the EMS personnel's relationship with the ACNP and other ED staff as well as the EMS personnel's assessment of the capabilities of the ACNP and the ED. Therefore, there is an economic benefit to maintaining good relationships with EMS providers.

Triage

Triage is a French word that means "to sort" and was originally applied to the sorting of grapes to be used in wine making. Triage in EDs denotes the process of assessing clients and prioritizing the order of care based on acuteness. All persons who present at an emergency room to seek care must be assessed by triage personnel. A variety of triage systems are used in EDs. These may range from a single level, comprehensive triage systems to a tiered system in which the client is assessed by two or more health care providers before an acuteness rating is assigned. Triage systems have a minimum of three acuteness categories, but some have five or more. Although a comprehensive discussion of triage systems is beyond the scope of this chapter, three basic acuteness categories are shared by the majority of triage systems. They are emergent, urgent, and nonurgent. Emergent designates patients who need care immediately; patients with conditions threatening life, limb, or special senses. Patients categorized as urgent need to be seen quickly, usually within 30 to 60 minutes of their arrival. Examples of conditions in the urgent category include abdominal pain, asthma exacerbations, and compound fractures or fractures with neurovascular compromise. The nonurgent category includes any complaint that can wait indefinitely for assessment and treatment in the clinically stable patient. Sore throats, simple fractures without neurovascular compromise, sunburns, earaches, simple lacerations, and foreign bodies in body cavities are usual conditions in the nonurgent category. Triage categories are dynamic. After clients are initially placed in a triage category, they are reassessed periodically to determine if their condition has changed sufficiently to affect the time frame in which they require care. Assessment of patients and assignment of a triage category generally requires the expertise of an experienced emergency care provider, most often the emergency nurse. Although ACNPs probably will not be assigned to the triage area, they must be familiar with the principles of triage and the meanings of each triage category. The ACNP may be called upon by the triage nurse to help decide which triage category is most appropriate for a particular client. Also, the ACNP may provide feedback to the triage nurse about the appropriateness of a triage category that has been assigned to a particular patient.

A notable exception to the triage process described above occurs during disaster situations. During a disaster, the ED may be confronted with an influx of patients in a relatively short period of time. Disaster triage differs significantly from routine triage. As in wartime, the emphasis in a disaster is the use of available resources, including personnel, to provide the most help to the largest number of patients. Priority care is given to patients who are critical but have a reasonable chance of survival. Critical patients who are not expected to survive are not treated until other clients are stabilized. Since ACNPs possess advanced assessment and treatment skills, they will probably be called upon to triage during a disaster. In addition to assigning patients to triage categories, the ACNP will probably be required to help coordinate care and assign patients to appropriate care areas. Finally, during a disaster, the ACNP may be required to provide care to patients who have been triaged.

Fast Track

Fast Track, or a similar name, is given to a section of the ED devoted exclusively to the rapid assessment, treatment, and disposition of uncomplicated patients. Using protocols and specific criteria, the triage nurse generally assigns the patients to be seen in the fast track. Usually located within or near the main ED, the fast track provides care for patients with conditions that could typically be handled in a primary care setting. The goals of fast tracks include decompression of patient flow in the main ED, reduced patient waiting time, and increased customer satisfaction. In addition to providing immediate care to these clients, those working the fast track usually refer the patient to an appropriate primary care provider in the community. Fast tracks may be open 24 hours each day but typically are only open during peak times of emergency department use, such as evenings and weekends. They are often staffed by midlevel providers, such as a nurse practitioner, and emergency nurses or unlicensed assistive personnel. Although a growing number of hospitals use midlevel providers in the main ED, some hospitals allow them to practice only in fast track settings.

Shock-Trauma

Most EDs have one or more rooms specially equipped to care for the most seriously ill patients. Generally known as shock-trauma, crash, or major rooms, these areas are typically larger than other rooms in the ED and are set up to provide immediate resuscitation and stabilization for critically ill patients. In the shock-trauma area, the ACNP functions as part of the multidisciplinary team. Ideally each member of the trauma or resuscitation team is assigned specific tasks before a patient arrives. The trauma or resuscitation team is usually led by the attending emergency medicine physician or trauma surgeon. Tasks that the ACNP may perform are the secondary assessment, a more thorough head-to-toe assessment completed after initial stabilization, and high-skill diagnostic and therapeutic procedures. These procedures may include endotracheal intubation, cricothyrotomy, chest tube insertion, diagnostic peritoneal lavage, and insertion of central vascular access devices. Once the patient is stabilized, the ACNP may perform other less urgent procedures such as suturing minor lacerations and stabilizing fractures. The ACNP may manage the patient's care while the patient is awaiting transfer to an inpatient area and may accompany the patient to the receiving unit in order to enhance continuity of care. If the patient is to be transferred to a facility offering speciality or a higher level of care, the ACNP may accompany and manage the patient during the transfer.

Chest Pain Centers

A growing number of EDs are adding specialized areas for the assessment, diagnosis, and treatment of chest pain. These chest pain centers (CPCs) have developed in response to the recommendations for rapid treatment of acute myocardial infarction (AMI). Additionally, most CPCs provide comprehensive assessment of chest pain not caused by an AMI, often allowing the patient to be discharged directly from the ED. This prevents many admissions, often to ICU. The role of the ACNP in the CPC may vary widely. Since most CPCs are currently located in larger, often teaching, hospitals, the ACNP will probably work collaboratively with a physician. Once patients begin treatment for AMI, the ACNP may manage their care until they are transferred to an inpatient unit.

Main Emergency Departments

For patients who do not meet the criteria for care in one of the specialty areas just discussed, care will be provided in the main ED. The main ED may have a trauma designation by the American College of Surgeons as a Level I, II, or III facility. Typically, a Level I trauma center is associated with a university and serves as a teaching facility that supports medical education and research in trauma. Moreover, there are physicians in house who can provide comprehensive care and services. A Level II facility is usually a community-based hospital that uses private physicians in house and on call speciality physicians. A Level III hospital is generally a rural facility or neighborhood-based facility that provides assessment and resuscitation followed by interhospital transfer of patients who are severely injured (Neff & Kidd, 1993). Hospitals that do not meet these criteria carry an implied designation as a Level IV trauma care hospital (Cardona, Hurn, Mason, Scanlon-Schilpp, & Veise-Berry, 1988).

Whether or not the main ED has a trauma designation, areas or rooms of the main ED are often used for specific conditions or age groups. For example, there may be an area with a dental chair designed for providing care to persons with eye, ear, nose, and throat conditions, and there may be a gynecology room equipped for doing pelvic examinations, collecting evidence from a female survivor of an alleged sexual assault, or assisting in a spontaneous vaginal delivery. Some EDs also have a specialized area for care of pediatric patients. The role of the ACNP may vary widely in the main ED, from providing care to any person in the main ED to providing services only for selected areas. Factors that may determine the role of the ACNP include location of the hospital, staffing, volume of patients, and severity of problems.

PEOPLE WHO SEEK CARE IN EMERGENCY DEPARTMENTS

Users of the Emergency Department

Identifying the users of emergency services provides information about the characteristics of individuals to whom the ACNP will be providing services. A national multisite study was conducted in 1995 and 1996 by the 1995 Research Committee of the Emergency Nurses Association (Cole, Bernardo, MacLean, Bayley, Lenaghan, & Manton, 1996). A total of 89 sites from 34 states throughout the United States participated in this study, designed to develop a profile of users of emergency services. Of the 89 EDs participating, the majority ($n = 66$) were not for profit. Although 87 provided general emergency services, 2 sites provided only pediatric services. Thirteen of the participating sites were rural, 12 were suburban, and 64 were urban. Twenty sites were verified by the American College of Surgeons or received state verification as a Level I trauma center; 16 were Level II; and 2 each were Level III and Level IV. The remaining 49 sites were not verified as trauma centers. As shown in

TABLE 9.2 Annual Emergency Department Visits as Reported by 89 Hospitals From 34 States Who Participated in the National Multi-site Research Project Conducted by the Research Committee of the Emergency Nurses Association (Cole et al., 1996)

Number of visits	Number of EDs reporting
0–5,000	1
5001–10,000	2
10,001–20,000	16
20,001–30,000	21
30,001–40,000	19
40,001–50,000	10
50,001–100,000	19
100,001 or greater	1

Table 9.2, the majority of EDs had annual visit rates of more than 21,001. The number of ED beds ranged from 5 to 50, with a mean of 20.20.

Data were reported for a total of 12,422 visits at the 89 sites. Visits were nearly evenly divided between females (50.1%) and males (49.9%) with a mean age of 35.4 years (SD = 24.1). As shown in Table 9.3, the majority of patients were White and single. Of the individuals with a stated religion, the majority were Protestant. The majority of patients arrived in the ED ambulatory ($n = 9348$), whereas 2,236 arrived by ambulance, 14 by helicopter, and 64 by police and 760 arrived by unknown means.

Conditions Treated

The health-care problems that compel patients to seek care in the ED are numerous and varied. It must be remembered that some individuals chose to come to the emergency department to seek care, whereas some people, such as someone undergoing cardiopulmonary resuscitation, are brought to the ED by others. Being aware of the types of health-care problems that people present with in the ED highlights the types of conditions that the ACNP will be assessing, diagnosing, and treating. As is often the case, the presenting reason for a visit is not always the final diagnosis. Table 9.4 provides the data for the 20 most frequent primary reasons for seeking care in the ED, and Table 9.5 identifies the top 20

TABLE 9.3 Demographic Characteristics of Users of Emergency Services as Reported by 89 Hospitals From 34 States Who Participated in the National Multi-site Research Project Conducted by the Research Committee of the Emergency Nurses Association (Cole et al., 1996)

Characteristic	Response	Frequency
Religion	Catholic	1861
	Jewish	128
	Protestant	2145
	Islamic/Muslim	21
	No religious preference	1374
	Unknown	6893
Marital status	Single	6455
	Married	3845
	Divorced/Separated	806
	Widowed	786
	Unknown	530
Race	Caucasian	7153
	African American	2060
	Asian/Pacific Islander	179
	Native American	36
	Hispanic	810
	Unknown	2185

discharge diagnoses. Note that the primary reason for seeking care in the ED is often not consistent with the discharge diagnosis. For example, the most common reason for seeking care is fever ($n = 566$), whereas the most common primary diagnosis is middle ear infection ($n = 562$). With so many nonurgent conditions treated in the ED, it is easy to lose sight of the fact that, regardless of the presenting complaint or the discharge diagnosis, people choose to seek care in the ED because they believe that their condition needs immediate attention.

ACUTE CARE NURSE PRACTITIONER PRACTICE IN THE EMERGENCY DEPARTMENT

Arrangements for practice will vary among EDs. The ACNP may be employed to provide services in the main ED or in a subdepartment, such as an urgent care or fast track clinic. In these types of clinics, the ED physician provides medical support to the ACNP. The nurse practi-

TABLE 9.4 Top 20 Reasons for Seeking Care in the ED as Reported by 89 Hospitals From 34 States Who Participated in the National Multi-site Research Project Conducted by the Research Committee of the Emergency Nurses Association (Cole et al., 1996)

Chief Complaint (CC)	Number of people with CC
Fever	566
Chest pain	561
Abdominal pain	481
Fall	416
Earache	362
Shortness of breath	342
Upper extremity laceration	316
Cough	297
Headache	292
Motor vehicle crash	270
Vomiting	265
Back pain	248
Labored breathing	204
Sore throat	204
Facial laceration	189
Hand/finger injury	172
Vertigo	166
Nausea	148
Neck pain	145
Low back pain	144

tioner, however, is often the only person to assess, diagnosis, and treat the patient.

When the ACNP is employed to provide services in the main ED, the most common arrangement is for the nurse practitioner to work alongside the ED physician. In this situation, the ACNP provides care to the next person to be seen irrespective of the triage designation. For example, if the physician is providing services to a patient and the next person to be seen is experiencing a myocardial infarction, the ACNP will assume the care for this person. Some physicians, however, prefer to provide care to the more critically ill patient while permitting the nurse practitioner to care for patients with nonurgent and urgent conditions. Working along side the physician allows for immediate consultation if needed.

The ACNP may also be employed as the sole provider in an ED.

TABLE 9.5 Top 20 Discharge Diagnoses of Patients Treated in the ED as Reported by 89 Hospitals From 34 States Who Participated in the National Multi-site Research Project Conducted by the Research Committee of the Emergency Nurses Association (Cole et al., 1996)

Diagnosis (DX)	Number of People with DX
Middle ear infection	562
Chest pain	320
Acute upper respiratory infection	289
Abdominal pain	271
Gastroenteritis	235
Viral pharyngitis	233
Open wound, finger	221
Asthma	211
Pneumonia	198
Urinary tract infection	175
Bronchiolitis	172
Chlamydial infection	169
Sprain, back	160
Bronchitis, acute	140
Sprain, foot & ankle	133
Headache	128
Contusion, chin	127
Canceled surgical procedure	121
Congestive heart failure, acute	111
Open wound, hand	101

Although this arrangement is less common, it can be used efficiently and effectively in rural EDs. One graduate from the Emergency/Ambulatory Care Nurse Practitioner program at the University of Texas Health Science Center at Houston is employed as a sole practitioner in a rural ED. This practitioner provides care to everyone who presents to the ED. Telephone consultation with a designated community physician is available at all times. Obviously, the responsibility associated with the role of sole practitioner is greater than working alongside the physician.

SKILLS NEEDED

When dealing with life and death situations, the ability to perform technical skills for the assessment, diagnosis, and management of these conditions is paramount. Technical skills are also important for assessment, diagnosis, and management of less severe conditions, such as joint aspiration, lumbar punctures, splinting, and nerve blocks. The technical skills that the nurse practitioner may be required to perform depending on the practice arrangement are listed in Table 9.1.

EMERGENCY DEPARTMENT SPECIFIC CONSIDERATIONS

There are many aspects of providing health care in an ED that are unique to the setting. Initial management and stabilization of conditions such as acute myocardial infarction and multiple trauma are unique to EDs. Drug overdose, suicide attempts, and alleged sexual assaults are other conditions that are specific to EDs. Additionally, many patients who present to the ED must have their initial diagnosis determined. This is in opposition to other areas of the hospital, where the patient has been admitted, the diagnosis has already been determined, and the ACNP is responsible for long-term management.

Although the ACNP may treat a particular patient more than once while employed in the ED, typically the care provided is of an acute, episodic nature. For example, rarely, if ever, is a patient started on insulin in the ED and then followed by the nurse practitioner in the ED for management. Rather, the individual is given a referral to a primary care physician in the community or clinic for initial and follow-up management. More commonly, the ACNP will encounter diabetic patients when they present with diabetic ketoacidosis or hyperosmolar hyperglycemic nonketosis, at which time they are stabilized and admitted. The same situation is true for patients with hypertension; the ACNP will manage these patients when they present with hypertensive crisis.

Often the initial presentation of the person in the ED is the only opportunity the ACNP will have to provide care to this person. The ACNP cannot assume that the patient will follow up with a community provider as directed; therefore, definitive care should be provided. For example, a suspected or confirmed streptococcal pharyngitis is often treated with an injection of penicillin rather than with a prescription for a course of oral penicillin. Suspected cases of gonococcal infection or pelvic inflammatory disease are often treated with an injection of ceftriaxone.

Because the ED may be the only department with in-house medical coverage at all times, the ACNP may be called upon to provide medical assistance to other areas of the hospital. It often happens that the emergency room ACNP or physician must respond to all cardiopulmonary resuscitations in the hospital and direct the resuscitation efforts while the private physician is en route.

Patients who are treated in the ED have three options for disposition. They can be discharged from the ED, admitted to an inpatient unit, or admitted to a 23-hour observation unit. The decision to admit to an inpatient or 23-hour observation unit can be very important because third party payors reimburse at different rates based on type of admission. Although the ACNP may face pressure to discharge a patient in order to conserve costs, the decision must be weighed against potential consequences for the patient if aftercare instructions are not followed. The ACNP should consult established criteria for admission or discharge for particular conditions to ensure that adequate treatment has been provided.

SUMMARY

This chapter has reviewed aspects of practice for the ACNP in the ED setting. Specific roles of the ACNP will vary depending on the ED setting (rural vs. urban), staffing, volume of patients seen, patient acuity, and practice arrangement (triage, fast track, shock-trauma, or main ED speciality areas). The ED provides the ACNP with an expanded scope of practice that includes ambulatory care through trauma care. As healthcare changes continue to occur, practice opportunities for the ACNP in the ED setting will continue to evolve.

REFERENCES

Cardona, V.D., Hurn, P.D., Mason, P.J.B., Scanlon-Schilpp, A.M., & Veise-Berry, S.W. (1988). *Trauma nursing: From resuscitation through rehabilitation.* Philadelphia: W. B. Saunders.

Cole, F.L., Bernardo, L., MacLean, S., Bayley, E., Lenaghan, P., & Manton, A. (1996). *LUNAR: Learning and using new approaches to research, a description of consumers of ED services.* Unpublished data.

Hardy, V.G.S. (1978). The emergency nurse practitioner: The role and training of an emerging health professional. *Journal of the American College of Emergency Physicians, 7,* 372–376.

Hayden, M.L., Davies, L.R., & Clore, E.R. (1982). Facilitators and inhibiters of the emergency nurse practitioner role. *Nursing Research, 31,* 294–299.

Haglund, C., & Dowling, W. (1993). The hospital. In S. Williams & P. Torrens (Eds.), *Introduction to health services* (4th ed.) (pp. 135–176). Albany, NY: Delmar.

Kovner, A.R. (1995). *Jonas's health care delivery in the United States.* New York: Springer.

MacPhail, E. (1992). Overview of emergency nursing and emergency care. In S.B. Sheehy (Ed.), *Emergency nursing: Principles and practice* (3rd ed.) (pp. 3–8). St. Louis: Mosby.

National Academy of Sciences, National Research Council (1966). *Accidental death and disability: The neglected disease of modern society.* Washington, DC: US Government Printing Office.

Neff, J.A., & Kidd, P.S. (1993). *Trauma nursing: The art and science.* St. Louis: Mosby.

SUGGESTED READINGS

Harwood-Nuss, A., & Luten, R.C. (1995). *Handbook of emergency medicine.* Philadelphia: J.B. Lippincott.

Pfenninger, J.L., & Fowler, G.C. (1994). *Procedures for primary care physicians.* St. Louis: Mosby.

Roberts, J.R., & Hedges, J.R. (1991). *Clinical procedures in emergency medicine* (2nd ed.). Philadelphia: W.B. Saunders.

Rosen, P. (1992). *Emergency medicine: Concepts and clinical practice.* St. Louis: Mosby.

Rund, D.A. (1996). *Essentials of emergency medicine.* St. Louis: Mosby.

10

An Evolving Critical Care Acute Care Nurse Practitioner Role: The Pulmonary Acute Care Nurse Practitioner and the Management of Patients Requiring Prolonged Ventilation

Suzanne M. Burns

Numerous roles for the acute care nurse practitioner (ACNP) in the intensive care unit (ICU) exist (Kleinpell, 1997), yet a dominant theme related to ACNP role implementation appears to be that of replacing residents and fellows in institutions where such positions are being "cut-back" (Hravnak, Rosenzweig, & Baldisseri, 1996; Lorenz, 1994; Mallison, 1993; Mitchell-DiCenso et al., 1996; Snyder et al., 1994; Spisso, O'Callaghan, McKennan, & Holcroft, 1990). In my own institution, neonatal nurse practitioners have only recently been hired as "house-staff" replacements; to date no other similar applications are projected. Although clear that this use of an ACNP may be very effective, some question how to implement the roles in other important advanced practice domains, such as teaching and research.

Another frequently mentioned role for the ACNP is that of "case manager," especially for patient populations that are complex, chronically ill, or costly for institutions (AJN Newsline, 1994; Anderson, 1997; Moore, 1993). In this model, other domains of advanced practice may emerge more consistently; the unique ability of the ACNP (to diagnose and treat the patient) is less dominant, however. Although care is "managed" by virtue of the fact that protocols and critical pathways delineate best practice and allow the case manager some autonomy in implementing such interventions, in most cases the clinician must work through the team to obtain orders and change practice. Unfortunately, this system is often bogged down by data collection and the complexity and burdensome nature of existing systems.

Both uses of an ACNP (i.e., house staff replacement or the case or outcomes manager) have merit, and aspects of each are appealing. They are existing roles, however, that an ACNP may conveniently occupy rather than unique positions developed specifically to take advantage of the unique constellation of an ACNP's knowledge and skills.

As noted, additional concerns surround the decreased valuing of traditional advanced practice functions such as teaching, consultation, research, and systems change. Although the ACNP is considered an advanced practitioner, the functional and focused nature of patient management may preclude the clinician's ability to regularly employ other advanced practice domains. In many institutions, the traditional clinical nurse specialist (CNS) role has been redesigned into such roles as case manager, leaving many wondering whether any "advanced clinicians" will be left to provide the important functions mentioned above.

In our medical ICU (MICU) we have developed the role of a full-time pulmonary "outcomes manager" (P-ACNP) for patients requiring long-term mechanical ventilation. The focus of the role is to progress care and improve the outcomes of these complex patients by systematically and comprehensively managing care. In addition to care management, the P-ACNP's role in the MICU includes staff development, clinical research, and involvement in institutional system changes. To date, the response to this model has been quite positive, since both quality and cost outcomes have been favorable. This chapter describes the role of the MICU P-ACNP and the emerging role of a rotating, "attending P-ACNP" in other critical care units as well.

EVOLUTION OF THE ROLE OF MICU P-ACNP

The care of patients who require long-term mechanical ventilation has long been the focus of work in our MICU. To that end, we have created numerous educational, clinical, and research initiatives and continue to do so in order to attain positive patient outcomes. These initiatives have also assumed institutional importance because the care of these patients is quite expensive.

Our work began with the development of the Burns Wean Assessment Program (BWAP) (Burns, Barton, Fahey, & Slack, 1991), a comprehensive weaning assessment program designed to help clinicians systematically evaluate, plan care for, and track the progress of long-term mechanically ventilated patients. Although related research (Burns, Burns, & Truwit, 1994) demonstrated the value of such a systematic assessment method, we recognized that consistent use of the program required that the process be standardized. Thus, we developed a specialty-trained weaning team to manage the patients. (Burns, Carpenter, Harris, & Bascle, 1995). The team approach was successful and was evaluated positively by members of the health-care team; the method, however, was somewhat cumbersome and inefficient because it required the regular coordination of team members to complete the assessments and care plans. In addition, team members often found it difficult to accomplish the evaluations, because they had patient assignments that often prevented "time away from the bedside" to complete assessments on patients other than those to which they were assigned.

To improve on these approaches, we designed and tested an "outcomes-managed" method of care delivery for this complex patient population. The design and results of this study are comprehensively described elsewhere (Burns et al., 1997); one outcome of the work is the permanent assignment of an ACNP with specialized expertise in the area of mechanical ventilation and weaning to the role of P-ACNP in the MICU. The MICU P-ACNP role, though still evolving, includes a wide variety of advanced practice role components. A description of the P-ACNP qualifications and role components follows.

ROLE DESCRIPTION FOR P-ACNP

Qualifications

The primary qualifications for this role are clinical expertise in the area of pulmonary nursing (specifically acute management of oxygenation and ventilation as well as weaning), a masters degree, and certification as an ACNP. Also required are a background in clinical teaching and research and excellent communications skills.

Clinical Management

The P-ACNP, in conjunction with the multidisciplinary team, is responsible for planning and coordinating the care of MICU patients who require prolonged ventilation. The goal of the P-ACNP is the attainment of positive patient, family, staff, and institutional outcomes.

Assessments done by the P-ACNP are complex and require that a wide variety of skills and a comprehensive knowledge base be used. For example, a typical weaning assessment may include completing a physical exam (lungs, heart, etc.); ordering and evaluating laboratory and radiographic data; performing arterial blood gas draws and assessment; calculating the BWAP (Burns et al., 1991), the Wean Index (Jabour, Rabil, Truwit, & Rochester, 1991), the rapid shallow breathing index (Yang & Tobin, 1991), and other standard weaning predictors (negative inspiratory pressure, positive expiratory pressure, etc.); and collecting a wide variety of data from patient care bedside "flow sheets" and monitoring systems (e.g., airway pressure monitoring and hemodynamic parameters). Although any of these elements separately may be accomplished or evaluated, or both, by select team members such as respiratory therapists or bedside nurses, the P-ACNP is able to independently perform and evaluate all; what results is an efficient, coordinated, comprehensive assessment.

In addition to accomplishing weaning-specific assessments, the P-ACNP functions as the "outcomes manager" for MICU ventilated patients. To that end, numerous elements of care designed to prevent complications, facilitate efficient movement through the system, and result in positive outcomes are evaluated and managed. The elements are identified by means of a clinical pathway (a.k.a., critical pathway) and include such factors as deep vein thrombosis prophylaxis, nutrition, mobility, and assignment to weaning trial protocols. Although medical house staff are always available to enter related orders (and it is preferred that they do so for educational purposes), the P-ACNP may facilitate the process by entering the orders as well. To date, the orders are a combination of those that do not require a physician's "verbal order" (e.g., nutrition consult, mobility, weaning assessments) and those that do (e.g., gut prophylaxis, deep vein thrombosis prophylaxis).

The P-ACNP assessments are discussed in daily multidisciplinary rounds, during which a plan of care is agreed upon. Finally, the P-ACNP writes the assessment and plan in the progress notes and coordinates the plan. This coordination of care is especially important when MICU weaning patients are "boarded" in other critical care units. In these cases, the P-ACNP often sees the patients long before the house staff (since teaching rounds are rarely completed until 11 a.m.). It is not unusual for the team to have up to 5 complex weaning patients boarded elsewhere, in addition to the 12 housed in the MICU. In these cases, the P-ACNP confers with the house staff related to care planning and implements the plans in the other units. This process is viewed very positively by the critical care unit staff in the other units because it facilitates care delivery and reduces the frustration of not having MICU house staff readily available.

Education and Development of Staff

The P-ACNP is integrally involved with the teaching of all clinicians working in the MICU (physicians, nurses, therapists, students, etc.). Much of the teaching is done daily in an informal manner (i.e., at bedside) and focuses on pulmonary-specific topics as well as a wide variety of other critical care areas (e.g., hemodynamics, lab interpretation). Other more formal presentations and teaching formats are a regular part of the role as well, however. For example, the P-ACNP regularly precepts staff and graduate students (both ACNP students and generic critical care students) in different aspects of advanced practice and expert pulmonary practice. In fact, the clinical teaching model at times assumes aspects of an apprenticeship, in which a clinician spends concentrated periods of time learning to master an area of practice under the tutelage of a "master." These "precepted" experiences are highly valued and requests for time with the P-ACNP are many (from outside as well as inside the institution). Formal presentations (especially on mechanical ventilation and weaning) are provided for nurses, respiratory therapists, physical therapists, physicians, and others both within the unit and outside of the unit.

Although the focus of the P-ACNP is the weaning patient, the broad ACNP (generalist) knowledge combined with an expert critical care repertoire of knowledge and skills makes the P-ACNP a powerful role model for less-seasoned individuals. Furthermore, the P-ACNP's background in diagnostic reasoning lends well to the development of critical decision-making skills in others.

Patient and family teaching primarily focuses on helping involved persons understand the weaning process and facilitating appropriate follow-ups once the patient is more stable. For the most part, the teaching is, of necessity, focused on the immediate information needs of patient and family in the MICU. Regardless, the P-ACNP often facilitates and/or coordinates future educational endeavors as well. An example is the patient with a substance abuse problem. Although clearly thc patient may not be ready to be counseled while in the ICU, the P-ACNP facilitates educational needs by attaining a "substance abuse consultation" at that time.

Clinical Research

MICU clinical research is collaborative and multidisciplinary and integrated into daily practice routines. The role of the P-ACNP includes a wide variety of research initiatives. Some of the projects fall into the category of quality improvement activities; some emerge from questions related to practice routines or interventions. For example, the P-ACNP regularly tracks "best practice indicators" (i.e., multidisciplinary standards of practice) by means of the clinical pathway. If it is identified that a negative outcome, such as an increase in urinary tract infections, occurs, the P-ACNP will evaluate the relationship of the increased infection rate to urinary catheter duration and catheter removal practices. In another pulmonary specific example, the P-ACNP may initiate a study to test the efficacy of weaning trial protocols. The P-ACNP often guides these projects and works with other members of the multidisciplinary team to improve practice.

The philosophy of the MICU related to clinical research is that research is considered "part of what we do" versus a special activity or a separate role. As a result, a major focus of the P-ACNP's role related to clinical research is as a mentor to less-seasoned researchers. Interest and participation in "research projects" is very high in the MICU, and our high productivity in the area is unique when compared with other critical care units within the institution and nationally. The P-ACNP plays an integral role in the development and nurturing of the MICU's research-based practice.

Systems Change

Although the dominant focus of the P-ACNP role is care management of patients requiring prolonged ventilation, it is in fact a dramatic and innovative system change that does much to focus staff and institutional efforts in order to attain positive outcomes. In many care management models, the involvement of the care manager is limited to care coordination and data tracking. The MICU P-ACNP model, in comparison, is a means of changing or focusing care in an extremely effective way by working side-by-side with physicians and other caregivers in order to effect real change by direct methods. In this model, P-ACNP "manages" the patients yet also performs many other essential elements of advanced practice.

FUTURE EVOLUTION OF MICU P-ACNP ROLE

Given the prominent role of the current P-ACNP in the MICU, potential adaptations focus on the increased use of this clinician's diagnostic skills and the broadening of practice privileges. As noted earlier, the MICU P-ACNP's role already includes a variety of pulmonary-specific and general care interventions. The P-ACNP regularly teaches staff, guides clinical research, and works on system changes within the medicine region. Although the role is an effective one, there are skills and additional knowledge that may be used to the advantage of the patient and system. For example, the flow of patients into and out of the MICU is still impeded somewhat by the complexity of patient care and the duration of medical teaching rounds. Although rounds are essential for team care planning as well as for teaching house staff, the duration of the rounds (in part a reflection of the complexity of the patients) makes timely care delivery difficult. Unfortunately, it is common for care management decisions to be deferred until after rounds, which often means that diagnostic tests are done late in the day; decision making is delayed as a result. By broadening the practice privileges of the P-ACNP to include the management of select patients (i.e., those to be transferred out of the unit and to a different medical care team), the care of the patients may be enhanced. For example, transfer orders could be written and transfers more expeditiously accomplished. Furthermore, the MICU P-ACNP's nursing focus would be extremely helpful in teaching and guiding the floor nurses assigned to these complex patients. The ACNP would serve a "bridging" function between ICU and floor that has not traditionally existed, thus promoting a truly "seamless" care delivery model.

THE P-ACNP IN OTHER UNITS—THE "ATTENDING" ACNP

The care of weaning patients varies tremendously from unit to unit within the institution. Although most long-term weaning occurs in the MICU, the institution continues to lose money on patients who require prolonged ventilation in other units as well. Nursing experts in weaning clearly exist in the MICU, but they don't exist in other units, and interventions known to enhance weaning outcomes are not routinely shared between units. In fact, even simple techniques for improving outcomes in this population (e.g., mobilizing, nutrition) are not embraced in other units. Instead, patients who are difficult to wean are eventually transferred to the MICU for management after weaning attempts are unsuccessful. Unfortunately, these patients are often quite debilitated by the time they are transferred. Although educational sessions by other units are often requested, little clinical supervision or follow-up guidance is provided to the units by experts. Recently, at least two different service lines have developed, or are in the process of developing: "step-down" and "progressive care" units for patients who require prolonged ventilation. Problems associated with the care of these patients have recently emerged and include patient management as well as educational issues.

To address these institutional needs, we have proposed, and are in the process of testing, a P-ACNP model for use in other critical care units. Since the model will not require the P-ACNP to be permanently based in the unit but instead will be assigned on an intermittent basis (i.e., month or months at a time), we have borrowed the term "attending nurse," coined by Linda Aiken (1990) and will call this role the attending P-ACNP.

In this role, the focus of the P-ACNP is to serve as an invited clinical expert, teacher, role model, and consultant in the care and management of patients requiring prolonged ventilation. The role requires that the P-ACNP be based in the unit for the duration of the rotation. The P-ACNP's constant presence allows for clinical guidance of house staff, nurses, and therapists.

The model is one that requires both "buy-in" and collaboration on the part of physicians, nurses, and other health care providers. It is important then, that the role and practice privileges be clearly articulated. Thus, specific practice privileges are granted based on the expert's knowledge and skills. In the case of the P-ACNP, for example, practice privileges include ventilatory management, weaning, diagnostics (i.e., arterial blood gases, chest x-ray), routine laboratory orders, and drug management (i.e., anxiolytics, sedatives, narcotics, bronchodilators). The privileges also include skills and management areas that contribute to the team's efficiency while promoting the use of the ACNP's scope and depth of expertise. For example, the P-ACNP's participation in rounds in a surgical unit would serve to guide the team's knowledge of the patient requiring prolonged mechanical ventilation while also actually managing the chronic and all too common conditions (diabetes, hypertension, chronic obstructive pulmonary disease, etc.) that often exist in this chronically critically ill patient population (Daly, Rudy, Thompson, & Happ, 1991). This generalist ACNP knowledge combined with the expert knowledge of mechanically ventilated patients would be especially useful in highly specialized units such as neurological, coronary, and thoracic-cardiovascular ICUs, where of necessity care is predominantly focused on one system rather than on the constellation of systems and comorbid medical conditions that contribute to ventilator dependency.

In addition to the P-ACNP's role modeling and teaching while attending in other units, unit research may also be encouraged. The presence of the P-ACNP allows less seasoned clinicians to draw on the expertise of individuals in areas outside of their specialty. Since the existing advanced practice model at our institution focuses the advanced clinician's efforts at the unit or (more recently) service line level, clinical leadership has been unevenly developed throughout the institution. The attending P-ACNP model encourages the sharing of such leaders in a wide variety of ways. By crossing traditional care delivery barriers such as service lines or units, and focusing on the delivery of quality care to a select patient population wherever they are in the institution, a true system change has occurred. Once implemented, it is likely that other innovations will emerge as well. Additionally, exposing other ICUs to the ACNP role will go a long way toward demystifying the role. Education of others related to what the ACNP can do is essential if unique applications that benefit patients are to evolve.

THE MODEL: WHO SUPPORTS?

The MICU P-ACNP is fully supported financially by the MICU. Practice privileges are developed in collaboration with the MICU medical director. In the case of the rotating attending P-ACNP, practice privileges are specified by the unit medical directors in order to improve the care of patients requiring ventilation in their units. The role is supported by participating service lines but the reporting structure is a bit more complicated. The attending P-ACNP reports to the head of patient care services, the specific unit administrators or managers, and each ICU medical director. As with other innovative changes, this support structure is in the process of evolving.

SUMMARY

Although the described roles of the MICU P-ACNP and the rotating attending P-ACNP in critical care units may be unique to our institution, they are potential models for use in others as well. It is probable that practicing ICU ACNPs may already be in similar roles, but it is important that we continue to test models that promote the unique abilities of the ACNP. It is likely that ACNPs will continue to be placed in house staff positions to fill gaps that exist and also to serve in case management or care-coordination positions. These are important and necessary roles and it is appropriate that ACNPs be used in them because they are well qualified to do so. We need not look solely to these existing roles as ICU-ACNP roles, however. Instead, it is important that we develop other roles as well, advanced practice roles that are inclusive of the knowledge and skills of the ACNP. The MICU P-ACNP and the rotating attending P-ACNP roles are designed to use the unique characteristics of an expert P-ACNP to focus the care of a very complex and often poorly managed patient population: those requiring prolonged mechanical ventilation. The roles focus on providing optimal care for the patient, regardless of the setting, while also recognizing the importance of managing patients in a cost-effective manner. Last, the roles integrate the domains of teaching and research while building on an already-existing collaborative partnership with our physician colleagues.

REFERENCES

Aiken, L.H. (1990). Charting the future of hospital nursing. *Image—The Journal of Nursing Scholarship, 22,* 72–78.

American Journal of Nursing Newsline. (1994, June). Acute care NPs chart a new career path for hospital RNs. *American Journal of Nursing, 69,* 72, 73.

Anderson, P. (1997). Managed care: Increased opportunities for acute care nurse practitioners. *AACN Clinical Issues, 8*(1), 101–107.

Burns, S.M., Barton, D., Fahey, S., Slack, D. (1991). Weaning from mechanical ventilation: A method for assessment and intervention. *AACN Clinical Issues in Critical Care Nursing, 2,* 372–387.

Burns, S.M., Burns, J.E., Truwit, J.D. (1994). Comparison of five clinical weaning indices. *American Journal of Critical Care, 3,* 342–352.

Burns, S.M., Marshall M., Burns, J.E., et al. (1998). Design, testing, and outcomes of an outcomes managed approach to patients requiring prolonged ventilation. *American Journal of Critical Care, 7,* 45–57.

Burns, S.M., Carpenter, R., Harris, R., & Bascle, M. Developing a team approach to weaning. (1995, May). *Nursing, 95,* 32TT–32WW.

Daly, B.J., Rudy, E.R., Thompson, K.S., & Happ, M.B. (1991). Development of a special care unit for chronically ill patients. *Heart & Lung 20,* 40–51.

Hravnak, M., Rosenzweig, M.Q., Baldisseri, M. (1996). Current questions with regard to acute care nurse practitioner preparation and role implementation. *AACN Clinical Issues, 7*(2), 289–299.

Jabour, E.R., Rabil, D.M., Truwit, J.D., Rochester, D.F. (1991). Evaluation of a new weaning index based on ventilatory endurance and the efficiency of gas exchange. *American Review of Respiratory Disease, 144,* 531–537.

Kleinpell, R.M. (1997). Acute-care nurse practitioners: Roles and practice profiles. *AACN Clinical Issues, 8*(1), 156–162.

Lorenz, B.T. (1994). Advanced practice nursing in the acute care setting. *Journal of Vascular Nursing XII*(4), 117–120.

Mallison, M.B. (1993). Nurses as house staff. *American Journal of Nursing, 93,* 7.

Mitchell-DiCenso, A., Guyatt, G., Marrin, et al. (1996). A controlled trial of nurse practitioners in neonatal intensive care. *Pediatrics, 98*(6), 1143–1148.

Moore, S.M. (1993). Promoting advanced practice nursing. *AACN Clinical Issues 4*(4), 603–608.

Snyder, J.V., Sirio, C.A., Angus, D.C., et al. (1994). Trial of nurse practitioners in intensive care. *New Horizons 2,* 296–304.

Spisso, J., O'Callaghan, C., McKennan, M., & Holcroft, J.W. (1990). Improved quality of care and reduction of house staff workload using trauma nurse practitioners. *Journal of Trauma 3*(6) 660–665.

Yang, K.L., & Tobin, M.J. (1991). A prospective study of indexes predicting the outcome of trials of weaning from mechanical ventilation. *New England Journal of Medicine, 324,* 1445–1450.

11

Expanding the Practice Opportunities for Acute Care Nurse Practitioners

Ruth M. Kleinpell and Carol Hudgins

The primary role of the Acute Care Nurse Practitioner (ACNP) is to provide health-care services across the continuum of acute care to patients who are acutely and critically ill (American Nurses Association, 1995). As the health-care environment changes, new opportunities for the ACNP are becoming increasingly available. Traditionally, nurse practitioners have provided services in the primary care setting, independent practices, and physician offices (Mirr, 1993; Sebas, 1994). Now more than ever, the ACNP is expanding the nurse practitioner roles into other settings. They are seen entering new arenas, such as bone marrow transplant, endocrinology, or oncology, and they are managing patients with a higher level of acuteness in hospital-based settings. This chapter will address the expansion of nurse practitioners into these new frontiers and issues that need to be addressed in order to ensure success in these new roles.

ACUTE CARE NURSE PRACTITIONER ROLES

ACNPs can practice in a variety of settings. The role of the ACNP in directing patient care includes comprehensive management, monitoring of complex therapies, high-risk interventions, and coordination of services. Whether the ACNP practices in the hospital, private practice, or emergency room, similar role functions can be seen. These include performing history and physical exams, appraising health risk, using diagnostic reasoning to formulate a plan of care, ordering and interpreting test results, performing indicated procedures and treatment, and consulting with and referring to other health-care professionals. An intrinsic component of the role is to optimize patient outcomes (American Nurses Association, 1995).

Although there may be basic similarities among ACNPs, there can be significant differences in the application of the role based on the specialty practice area. ACNPs practicing in the hospital setting may be located on a specific unit, where they manage the care of all patients admitted to the unit. The ACNP can also follow a specific type of patient, such as open heart, liver transplant, or pulmonary failure patients (Genet et al., 1995). In a specialty practice, the ACNP is hired by a physician or practice group. The scope of care may then cross the continuum of care from outpatient clinic to inpatient hospital responsibilities.

EXPANDING ACUTE CARE NURSE PRACTITIONER ROLES

Opportunities for expanding the practice settings for ACNPs will mean identifying potential practice arenas and meeting market demands with new and innovative roles. As the role of the ACNP evolves, it will be essential to be flexible. For example, a practicing ACNP related that although she was originally hired to work in a neurosurgical intensive care unit (ICU) to cover patients postoperatively, she often found that there was an overlap between her role and the role of the neurosurgical residents. The ACNP identified that a need existed on the step-down unit for a practitioner to coordinate patient care management and discharge planning. She moved into the new role, and the importance of her care became so evident that a second ACNP was soon hired to work in a similar capacity with patients transferred from the neurosurgical ICU to the general care areas.

Another ACNP was initially hired to work with a cardiology group covering patients post cardiac catheterization. Patients were routinely monitored overnight and then discharged the next day. The ACNP independently managed these patients using protocol orders, performing precatheterization and postcatheterization teaching, and planning for discharge. Her role was soon expanded to cover overflow patients from the coronary care unit, with a variety of cardiac-related diagnoses. When unit restructuring was done to accommodate increased patient census, two additional ACNPs were hired, and they now provide 7-days-a-week coverage of unit patients.

Another ACNP in practice with an interventional cardiologist was hired to help manage inpatients at two different hospitals. The comprehensiveness of her care enabled the cardiologist to expand his outpatient practice to include a cholesterol and coumadin clinic, which the ACNP now manages independently. In this role, the ACNP shares rounding responsibilities in one of the two hospitals, seeing all inpatients and collaboratively planning their care with the physician. The ACNP participates in evaluating inpatients for interventional studies and oversees stress tests, evaluating the patient's electrocardiogram, hemodynamic, and symptom responses during testing.

Coverage of clinic patients includes evaluating patients on follow-up visits, adjusting medications, and assessing the need for diagnostic or lab studies. In managing the cholesterol clinic, the ACNP evaluates lab screening studies, diet, exercise, and profile risk and determines the indicated treatment plan, including lifestyle changes, diet, medications, and return visit frequency. In managing the coumadin clinic, the ACNP evaluates coagulation study results and adjusts medication dosing. The role has truly evolved into a collaborative practice role, with the ACNP functioning as an independent practitioner in several aspects of the role.

These examples portray the evolving nature of ACNP practice. Once ACNPs are integrated within a practice site, role changes or expansion, or both, can provide new opportunities for ACNP practice. As described in chapter 1, ACNPs are moving into a variety of practice settings, including secondary and primary care areas. Often, these roles are newly created positions that the ACNP can help formulate to fit identified needs.

ESSENTIALS TO PRACTICE

Success in expanding the practice opportunities for ACNPs will depend on several factors. These opportunities include obtaining role recognition, dealing with resistance to the role, and combating barriers to practice. The role of the ACNP is only beginning to gain recognition. Practicing

ACNPs report that many physicians are unaware of, or feel threatened by, the ACNP role. Continued dissemination regarding the ACNP role and the role potential is needed to make physicians, health-care professionals, and health-care consumers aware of the existence of ACNPs.

Misperceptions exist that the ACNP role is only that of a physician extender. Although the literature on ACNP practice is growing, early reports that the ACNP was filling inpatient hospital needs that arose from decreases in medical resident and house staff coverage did portray the ACNP as performing physician substitution functions. Exposure to the comprehensive and coordinated care of the ACNP has helped to change the outlook of some practitioners; however, ACNPs cannot depend on personal experience or exposure to the role to result in rapid acceptance of ACNP practice. ACNPs must actively publicize the role, not only in terms of role capabilities but also in terms of role effectiveness and outcomes data.

Many ACNPs report resistance to the role from physicians and other health-care professionals, including nursing (Kleinpell, 1997). Uncertainty about the ACNP role and the belief that the ACNP is practicing medicine and not advanced practice nursing has led to role resistance. Confusion as to whether the ACNP role will replace the roles of clinical nurse specialists has also added to the resistance. Educating nurses on ACNP practice can facilitate acceptance of the role. Additionally, highlighting aspects of collaborative practice can assist in gaining support for the role from similar providers, including other nurse practitioner groups and physician assistants.

Combating barriers to practice, such as advanced practice nursing recognition in state nurse practice acts, gaining prescribing privileges, obtaining practice privileges, and deciphering reimbursement qualifications will continue to be challenges to ACNP practice. As the practice settings for ACNPs expand, other practice-related issues may arise that will pose threats to the practice capabilities of the ACNP. These barriers must be removed or lessened to allow the ACNP to function effectively. To help ensure role success, ACNPs must be legislatively active and participate in policy making at the state and federal levels.

GROWING NEED FOR ACNPS

The population is aging, with a consequential increase in the number of persons with chronic illnesses. Episodes of acute illness or exacerbation of chronic illness states will need to be managed and treated in efficient and effective ways if rising health-care costs are to be curtailed and optimal patient outcomes achieved. Stabilization of acute and chronic illness states is directly within the scope of practice of the ACNP, and the need for ACNPs to manage these patients in a variety of settings will only continue to expand.

The future is bright for the ACNP because it is a new and expanding career opportunity. The role of the ACNP will only continue to evolve as more ACNPs enter the marketplace and continue to extend practice boundaries in secondary and tertiary care settings. There will be ongoing challenges for the ACNP in the acute care setting, such as avoiding identification as a physician substitute and dealing with resistance to the role and restrictions on practice privileges. Demonstrating advanced clinical decision-making skills and providing comprehensive care will need to be performed on a consistent basis to help overcome such obstacles.

ACNPs will need to be creative and innovative in terms of identifying potential practice sites. Areas such as home care, same-day surgery centers, urgent care centers, subacute care facilities, and acute care clinics, in addition to hospital inpatient areas, hold potential for ACNP role development. Many practicing ACNPs report that their current positions were created by their employer, or they were approached by their employer to assist in the development of an ACNP role. The ability to actively participate in formulating aspects of the position has been cited as a distinct advantage of ACNP practice (Kleinpell, 1997).

Advanced practice nursing offers an exciting and challenging career, and the role of the ACNP offers nursing another opportunity to significantly impact health care and improve the quality of patient care and patient outcomes. The role will continue to evolve as nurse practitioners move into expanding acute care settings. Additionally, opportunities to formulate new roles for the ACNP will occur as ACNPs become a recognized and accepted member of the health-care team.

REFERENCES

American Nurses Association. (1995). *Standards of clinical practice and scope of practice for the acute care nurse practitioner.* Washington, DC: American Nurses Publishing.

Genet, C., Brennan, P., Ibgbotson-Wolff, S., et al. (1995). Nurse practitioners in a teaching hospital. *Nurse Practitioner, 20,* 47–54.

Kleinpell, R. (1997). Acute care nurse practitioners: Roles and practice profiles. *AACN Clinical Issues, 8,* 156–162.

Mirr, M. (1993). Advances in clinical practice: A reconceptualized role. *AACN Clinical Issues, 4,* 599–606.

Sebas, M. (1994). Developing a collaborative practice agreement for the primary care setting. *Nurse Practitioner, 19,* 49–51.

Index